The Electrocardiogram in Acute Myocardial Infarction

Edited by

Ian P. Clements, MD

Consultant
Division of Cardiovascular Diseases and Internal Medicine
Mayo Clinic and Mayo Foundation
Assistant Professor of Medicine
Mayo Medical School
Rochester, Minnesota

**Futura Publishing
Company, Inc.**
Armonk, New York

Library of Congress Cataloging-in-Publication Data

The electrocardiogram in acute myocardial infarction / edited by Ian
  P. Clements : with contributors.
     p. cm.
  Includes bibliographical references and index.
  ISBN 0-87993-693-2
  1. Myocardial infarction—Diagnosis. 2. Electrocardiography.
  I. Clements, Ian P.
  [DNLM: 1. Myocardial Infarction—diagnosis.
  2. Electrocardiography—methods. WG 300 E38 1998]
  RC685.I6E43 1998
  616.1′23707547—dc21
  DNLM/DLC
  for Library of Congress   97-50183
                                          CIP

Copyright © 1998
Mayo Foundation

Published by
Futura Publishing Company, Inc.
135 Bedford Road
Armonk, New York 10504

LC#: 97-50183
ISBN#: 0-87993-693-2

Printed in the United States of America.

Printed on acid-free paper.

List of Contributors

A. A. Jennifer Adgey, MD, FRCP, FACC
Professor, Consultant Cardiologist, Regional Medical Cardiology Centre, Royal Victoria Hospital, Belfast, Ireland

Yochai Birnbaum, MD
Department of Cardiology, Beilinson Medical Center, Petah-Tiqva; Sackler Faculty of Medicine, Tel Aviv University; Tel Aviv, Israel

Timothy F. Christian, MD
Senior Associate Consultant, Division of Cardiovascular Diseases and Internal Medicine, Mayo Clinic and Mayo Foundation; Associate Professor of Medicine, Mayo Medical School; Rochester, Minnesota

Ian P. Clements, MD
Consultant, Division of Cardiovascular Diseases and Internal Medicine, Mayo Clinic and Mayo Foundation; Assistant Professor of Medicine, Mayo Medical School; Rochester, Minnesota

Shahid Hameed, MRCP
Registrar in Cardiology, Regional Medical Cardiology Centre, Royal Victoria Hospital, Belfast, Ireland

Stephen C. Hammill, MD
Consultant, Division of Cardiovascular Diseases and Internal Medicine, Mayo Clinic and Mayo Foundation; Professor of Medicine, Mayo Medical School; Rochester, Minnesota

Mark T. Harbinson, MB, MRCP
Registrar in Cardiology, Regional Medical Cardiology Centre, Royal Victoria Hospital, Belfast, Ireland

Mitchell W. Krucoff, MD, FACC, FCCP
Director, Ischemia Monitoring Laboratory, Duke University Medical Center; Director, Cardiac Catheterization Laboratory, Durham Veterans Administration Medical Center; Durham, North Carolina

Manlik Kwong, BSE
Hewlett-Packard Corporation, Corvalis, Oregon

Stephen R. McMechan, MB, MRCP
Registrar in Cardiology, Regional Medical Cardiology Centre, Royal Victoria Hospital, Belfast, Ireland

Philip B. Oliva, MD
Visiting Scientist at the Division of Cardiovascular Diseases and Internal Medicine, Mayo Clinic and Mayo Foundation, Rochester, Minnesota

Karlton S. Pettis, MD
Research Associate, Department of Medicine, Division of Cardiology, Duke University Medical Center, Durham, North Carolina

Stephen J. Pieper, MD
Fellow in Cardiovascular Diseases, Mayo Graduate School of Medicine, Rochester, Minnesota

James E. Pope, MD, FACC
Research Associate Professor, Ischemia Monitoring Laboratory, Duke University Medical Center, Durham, North Carolina; Associate, HeartCare Institute of Tampa, Tampa, Florida

Samuel Sclarovsky, MD
Department of Cardiology, Beilinson Medical Center, Petah-Tiqva; Sackler Faculty of Medicine, Tel Aviv University; Tel Aviv, Israel

Maarten L. Simoons, MD, PhD, FESC, FACC
Professor of Cardiology, Thorax Center, Department of Cardiology, University Hospital "Dijkzigt," and Erasmus University Rotterdam, Rotterdam, The Netherlands

Rolf F. Veldkamp, MD, PhD
Fellow in Cardiology, Thorax Center, Department of Cardiology, University Hospital "Dijkzigt," and Erasmus University Rotterdam, Rotterdam, The Netherlands

Galen S. Wagner, MD
Associate Professor, Department of Medicine, Division of Cardiology, Duke University Medical Center, Durham, North Carolina

Foreword

The balance between the diagnostic and therapeutic aspects of any clinical entity tends to shift alternately between one or the other. Currently, our therapeutic ability to achieve and maintain reperfusion in patients with acute myocardial ischemia and infarction is greater than our clinical diagnostic ability. Our primary diagnostic method, the electrocardiogram (ECG), has potential for being a strong enough diagnostic tool to balance the therapeutic weight of either intravenous or intracoronary reperfusion methods. Strengths of the ECG include: 1) its almost universal availability in hospitals and its potential universal availability in emergency medical vehicles; 2) its potential for wireless transmission to minicomputers in the hands of the on-call cardiologist; 3) its inexpensiveness in our ever most cost-conscious medical community; 4) its provision of on-line diagnostic information; 5) its ability to reveal the presence of a myocardial current injury directed toward the region supplied by the culprit coronary artery; and 6) the proven quantitative relationship between the extent of the current of injury and the severity of myocardial ischemia.

What are the weaknesses of the standard ECG as a diagnostic method in acute myocardial ischemia and infarction? It is not new in a society that values the new; most physicians believe they know all there is to know about this ancient method. It provides a single "snapshot" in time, and efforts to popularize continuous ECG ischemia monitoring have failed to overcome the nuisance of false positivity due to skeletal muscle artifacts. The ECG is often falsely negative for indicating infarction caused by acute thrombosis of the left circumflex artery. However, the clinical impression of ECG false negativity is magnified because all patients with enzymatic evidence of myocardial infarction are considered the denominator rather than only those with acute thrombotic etiology. There also are insufficient clinical research studies to assess accurately the capability of the ECG to estimate the extent of acutely ischemic myocardium, to indicate the timing and extent of reperfusion, and to measure the amount of myocardium salvaged.

The cumulative result of these real and perceived weaknesses of the ECG creates its current underutilization. It is not obtained by paramedics on arrival. If obtained, it is not transmitted electronically to the on-call cardiologist. It is first obtained in the emergency department after an average time of 1 hour. Published quantitative methods for estimating the extent or timing of the ischemia/infarction process are neither calculated by automated commercial programs nor applied by clinicians. Continuous ECGs are not recorded during reperfusion therapy to determine effectiveness. Published methods for estimating salvage are not applied.

Ian P. Clements has accepted the clinically important task of bringing focus to correcting this diagnostic/therapeutic imbalance. Perhaps the addition of other leads or higher frequency signals or spatial relationships will be helpful. Perhaps future clinical research will identify more accurate formulas for calculating the extent of ischemia, reperfusion, and salvage. And hopefully, more appreciation of the information already available from this well-worn, faithful clinical companion will enhance physician decision-making support as our armament of therapeutic methods for managing patients with acute myocardial ischemia and infarction continues to expand.

Galen Wagner, MD
Duke University Medical Center
Durham, North Carolina

Preface

This monograph provides an up-to-date review of the use of the electrocardiogram in acute myocardial infarction. The descriptive electrocardiographic features associated with myocardial infarction are well known. However, now that interventional treatment such as acute thrombolysis and angioplasty is so successful in limiting evolving myocardial infarction, new roles for the electrocardiogram in acute infarction are being explored. Modification of the electrocardiographic recording technique, such as precordial electrocardiographic mapping, may lead to better diagnostic information. Other approaches, such as examination for fluctuation in electrocardiographic variables, may provide prognostic data.

An exceedingly valuable clinical role for the electrocardiogram is the detection of reperfusion in acute myocardial infarction. This is possible using continuous ST-segment monitoring with both the standard and vector electrocardiogram. These techniques are currently used in the clinical setting.

The electrocardiogram must provide diagnostic information. More detailed analysis of the standard electrocardiogram in acute myocardial infarction enables more diagnostic information to be derived from the electrocardiogram. This information is enhanced when it is cross-correlated with precise coronary artery anatomy and myocardial perfusion images in acute infarction.

It would be very beneficial if myocardial infarction could be quantified early in infarction. Furthermore, it would be of immense benefit if the effects of interventions could be quantified. Some aspects of the electrocardiogram may allow infarct quantification.

The electrocardiogram is invariably the first diagnostic test performed when acute myocardial infarction is suspected. The earlier the electrocardiogram is made available to the treating physician the better, because the therapeutic decisions can then be made much sooner. Thus, techniques to make the electrocardiogram available to the managing physician before the patient gets to the hospital are very important. In these circumstances, it is also necessary to understand the evolution of the early postinfarct electrocardiogram.

During the hospital phase of myocardial infarction, electrocardiographic monitoring is usual, and, in addition to detecting infarct-related artery reocclusion, the electrocardiogram may detect signs of impending left ventricular rupture. This event is now a major cause of mortality after acute myocardial infarction.

The electrocardiogram has a long history in cardiology, and with the revolution in treatment of myocardial infarction and the active interest in developing new electrocardiographic techniques in this setting, the electrocardiogram should remain an important evolving clinical tool.

I would like to thank my coauthors, the staff of the Section of Publications of the Mayo Clinic (O. Eugene Millhouse, PhD, Roberta J. Schwartz, Mary K. Horsman, and Dorothy Tienter), and, finally, Steven E. Korn of Futura Publishing Company Inc. for their expertise, encouragement, and support in the completion of this project.

Ian P. Clements, MD

Dedication

To Deirdre, Áine, and Sinéad.

Table of Contents

1

Continuous Multilead ST-Segment Monitoring in Acute Myocardial Infarction

Rolf F. Veldkamp, MD, PhD
Maarten L. Simoons, MD, PhD, FESC, FACC
James E. Pope, MD, FACC
Mitchell W. Krucoff, MD, FACC, FCCP

Introduction

Patients who have acute myocardial infarction with early, complete, and stable reperfusion after thrombolytic therapy have a favorable prognosis. Patients without early and stable reperfusion through the infarct-related artery may benefit from further pharmacologic or mechanical revascularization interventions. The most reliable method for assessing perfusion status of the infarct-related artery is repeated coronary angiography. However, this is a burden on patient and hospital resources, and catheterization laboratory facilities are not available at all hospitals. Therefore, a reliable noninvasive assessment technique capable of detecting reperfusion and reocclusion over time would be useful. Recently, continuously updated ST-segment recovery analysis has been shown to be accurate for real-time noninvasive assessment of vessel patency.[1-4] Various multilead continuous ST-segment monitoring systems, or ST monitors, have been developed and are available commercially.[5-10] This chapter describes the application of these ST monitors during acute myocardial infarction.

From: Clements, IP (ed). *The Electrocardiogram in Acute Myocardial Infarction.* Armonk, NY: Futura Publishing Company, Inc. © Mayo Foundation 1998.

Physiology

Approximately 75% of patients with acute myocardial infarction have ST-segment changes suggesting transmural ischemia at presentation (presumably new ST-segment elevation or depression $\geq$ 1 or 2 mm), but this percentage may increase with serial electrocardiographic (ECG) assessments.[11–13] Patients without ST-segment deviation generally have smaller infarcts and often receive less benefit from reperfusion therapy.[13–17] Without reperfusion of the infarct-related artery, the ST deviation gradually lessens over the next few hours because of necrosis of the myocytes and, thus, loss of myocardial mass ("burn out").[12,18–20] After reperfusion, a more rapid normalization of the ST segment occurs.

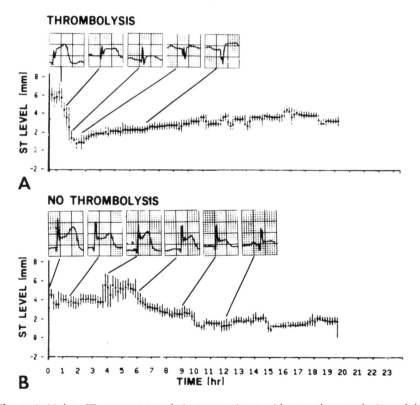

Figure 1. Holter ST-segment trends in two patients with complete occlusion of the infarct-related artery. **A.** Successful reperfusion after intracoronary thrombolysis is characterized by the sudden decline of ST-segment elevation. **B.** Unsuccessful reperfusion with a slow, gradual achievement of ST steady state. (Reproduced with permission from Reference 20.)

This phenomenon has been demonstrated clearly during intracoronary administration of thrombolytic drugs to dissolve the thrombus occluding the infarct-related artery.[18-20] The differences in ST-segment behavior over time during continuous coronary occlusion and after reperfusion through the infarct-related coronary artery are shown in Figure 1.

Hackett et al[21] demonstrated, in 45 patients with acute myocardial infarction, the close temporal relationship between ST-segment elevation and coronary artery occlusion before and after intracoronary infusion of streptokinase, using continuous ST-segment Holter monitoring with concomitant serial angiographic observations. Fifteen patients had 29 episodes of transient ST-segment normalization: 12 episodes (in 8 patients) occurred spontaneously before coronary angiography and 17 (in 8 patients) during coronary catheterization, of which 13 (in 7 patients) occurred during streptokinase infusion. Occlusion was always found during episodes of ST-segment elevation, and patency coincided with resolution of ST-segment elevation (Figure 2). Coronary reperfusion in the early phase of myocardial infarction was frequently intermittent and was reflected by ST-segment recovery and reelevation. The percentages of patients with ST evidence of intermittent reperfusion in seven different studies are listed in Table 1.[1,8,21-25] Although different therapies aimed at reperfusion were applied, intermittent reperfusion was observed consistently in approximately 37% of the patients (95%

Table 1

Occurrence of Intermittent Reperfusion in Acute Myocardial Infarction Reported in Seven Different Studies

Author	No. of Patients	Treatment	A/ST	Intermittent Reperfusion No. of Patients	%	Before Treatment No. of Patients	%
Davies et al[22]	9	IC-SK	A + ST	6	67	1	11
Hackett et al[21]	45	IC-SK	A + ST	22	49	8	21
Krucoff et al[1]	22	IV-TTX/PTCA	A + ST	11	50	5	31
Dellborg et al[8]	103	rt-PA/placebo	ST	35	34	16	34*
Kwon et al[23]	31	IV-TTX	ST	11	35	Not reported	
Veldkamp et al[24]	82	IV-TTX	ST	32	39	Not reported	
Langer et al[25]	618	IV-TTX	ST	221	36	Not reported	
	910			338	37	30/110	27

A = Serial angiographic observations; IC-SK = intracoronary streptokinase; IV-TTX = intravenous thrombolytic treatment; rt-PA = recombinant tissue type plasminogen activator; ST = continuous ECG-ST-segment monitoring.

* In the placebo group.

(Reproduced with permission from Reference 59.)

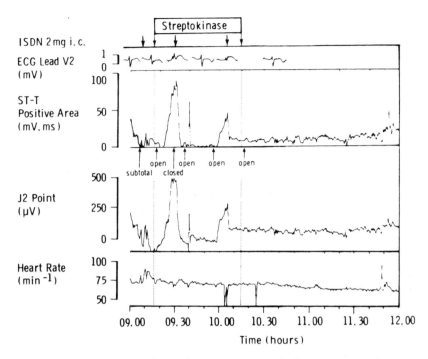

Figure 2. Computerized analysis of a continuous ambulatory ECG (Holter—ECG) from a patient with recurrent ST-segment elevation and coronary reocclusion during continuous infusion of streptokinase. Initially ST-segment elevation was recorded at 9:06 hours, and after intracoronary isosorbide dinitrate (ISDN), the ST segment returned to baseline. ST-segment elevation recurred with angiographically documented coronary occlusion at 9:30 hours during continuous infusion of streptokinase. After additional ISDN, the ST segment again returned to baseline, with angiographic documentation of coronary recanalization. ST-segment elevation recurred at 9:58 hours, but coronary angiography was not performed during this episode. After additional ISDN, the ST segment again returned to baseline. (Reproduced with permission from Reference 21.)

confidence interval, 34% to 40%), and 27% of the episodes of reperfusion (19% to 36%) occurred before either thrombolytic therapy or coronary angioplasty was initiated. Intermittent coronary reperfusion may be explained by the dynamics of thrombus formation and breakdown at the site of plaque rupture under influence of treatment with aspirin, heparin, thrombolytic agents, and vasodilators, or by coronary spasm or intermittent collateral blood supply.[1,8,21,22,26,27] It has been reported that patients with intermittent reperfusion, as evidenced by dynamic ST-segment changes, have a larger infarct size indicated by a higher maximal lactate dehydrogenase-1 level, a more pronounced change in

QRS vector after 24 hours, a longer time to peak level of creatine kinase, and a (nonsignificant) tendency toward a higher 1-year mortality than patients who do not have ST evidence of intermittent reperfusion.[8] In 618 patients of the Global Utilization of Streptokinase and Tissue Plasminogen Activator for Occluded Coronary Arteries (GUSTO-I) ECG substudy, a weak but significant inverse relationship was found between the presence of recurrent ST-segment elevation and left ventricular ejection fraction ($r = -0.16$, $P = 0.001$).[25] It is not known whether these unfavorable outcomes are caused by repeated reperfusion injury, longer period of total occlusion, or a higher incidence of lesions in more proximal coronary arteries, or whether this is largely due to intermittent reperfusion being more obvious when infarction generates higher ST-segment amplitudes. Although more studies of the pathophysiology and clinical relevance of intermittent reperfusion are needed, these data strongly suggest that cyclic reperfusion does have clinical significance regarding outcome and effect of treatment.

History of ST Monitoring

The observation of rapid ST-segment recovery at the moment of angiographically documented reperfusion led to studies that correlated quantitative ST-segment recovery with patency of the infarct-related artery. Several studies comparing ST-segment deviation between a post-treatment ECG, typically 60 to 180 minutes after the onset of thrombolytic treatment, and a fixed pretreatment reference ECG have been reported.[28-33] If the ST segment has recovered below a threshold expressed as a percentage of the pretreatment reference ECG ST level, reperfusion is considered to have occurred. If the ST segment did not recover below this threshold, reperfusion is considered to have failed.

Continuous ST monitoring with Holter recorders was developed to better document the timing of reperfusion. Recordings were analyzed retrospectively and used to distinguish patients with reperfused infarct-related arteries from those in whom the infarct-related artery failed to reperfuse after treatment.[20,21] However, Holter recordings are limited by the number of leads used, and they cannot be used at the bedside to guide clinical care because they require off-line analysis. Therefore, dedicated continuous multilead computerized ECGs have been developed by several groups to measure, compare, and display the ST segment in real time so that the recorded information can be used to guide clinical care.[5-10] The major application of these devices is the display of ST-segment recovery and of new ST-segment abnormalities as a reflection of ischemia in various unstable coronary syndromes, such as acute myocardial infarction, unstable angina pectoris, and post-coronary angioplasty. Accordingly, they have been called "ST monitors" or "ischemia monitors."

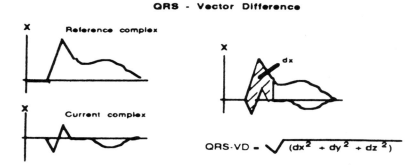

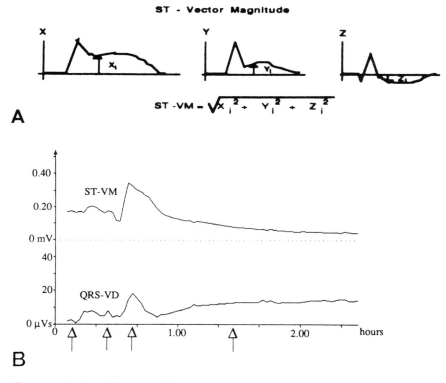

Figure 3. A. The definition of the QRS vector difference is displayed in the **upper panel**. The reference mean QRS complex at the start of the continuous recording and the current mean QRS complex in lead X of the orthogonal lead system are

General Principles of ST Monitoring

The ST Monitor

Two different approaches to dedicated continuous multilead computerized ECG have been developed and marketed to provide real-time information on the dynamic ECG changes at the bedside, with optional alarms warning a clinician when such changes occur. The first method is based on continuous sampling and averaging of the 12-lead ECG.[5,9,10] The averaged complexes are stored in memory together with digital measurements of the ST segment, typically measured 60 milliseconds after the J-point. Recorded ECGs and trends of ST-segment deviation over time in all 12 leads are accessible at the bedside or at a central monitoring station that displays the ST-segment recordings of many patients simultaneously. The second approach uses continuous recording of mean vector electrocardiography complexes computed from the Frank lead system.[6-8] These ST-monitoring systems are available as stand-alone units or the signal may be relayed to a central monitoring unit, displaying either the orthogonal leads or derived 12-lead ECGs. In acute myocardial infarction studies, the two derived variables most often followed over time are the QRS vector difference and the ST-vector magnitude (Figure 3), although many other vector-derived variables can

◀——————————————————————————————————

shown separately and plotted superimposed. The **hatched area**, dx, is the QRS vector difference in lead X. Accordingly, dy and dz are calculated. The root of the squares of dx, dy, and dz defines the QRS vector difference (QRS-VD) between the reference and the current ECG. The definition of the ST-vector magnitude of an orthogonal ECG is displayed in the **lower panel**. The **arrows** indicate the ST deviation 20 ms after the J-point in each of the three leads, assigned X_i, Y_i, and Z_i. The root of the square X_i, Y_i, and Z_i defines the ST-vector magnitude (ST-VM). **B.** Two trends show the change over time in the QRS-VD and ST-VM of a patient with myocardial infarction. The **first arrow** (from the left) indicates the first angiogram, which revealed an occluded left circumflex coronary artery despite intravenous administration of urokinase. Limited perfusion (TIMI grade 1 flow) was achieved with the guide wire. Subsequent balloon angioplasty resulted in TIMI grade 3 flow, indicated by the **second arrow**. The patient then had an episode of coronary spasm treated with intracoronary nitroglycerin, indicated by the **third arrow**. Approximately 50 minutes after reestablishment of coronary patency, the QRS changes reach a plateau, indicating the end of changes in the QRS morphology. Vectorcardiographic signs of reperfusion are the rapid changes in QRS-VD, with an early plateau and rapid decline of the ST-VM. Rapid decline of the ST-VM derived from the vectorcardiogram is similar to the rapid resolution of ST elevation seen in the conventional ECG at the moment of reperfusion. (A. Lower panel and B. reproduced with permission from Dellborg M, Topol EJ, Swedberg K: Dynamic QRS complex and ST-segment vectorcardiographic monitoring can identify vessel patency in patients with acute myocardial infarction treated with reperfusion therapy. *Am Heart J* 122:943–948, 1991.)

be calculated and displayed over time.[7,8] The QRS vector difference is especially sensitive to changes in the QRS morphology and duration, making it a variable that reflects infarct evolution and conduction changes. The ST-vector magnitude is the result of the ST-segment deflection in the three orthogonal leads and, thus, reflects the presence or absence of ST-segment deviation as a result of ischemia, similar to the recording of the ST-segment deviation in the 12-lead device.

Other devices that may be used for ST monitoring are arrhythmia-monitoring systems and Holter recorders. ECG monitoring systems used to detect cardiac arrhythmias in real time are available in most coronary care units, intensive care units, medium care or step-down units (telemetry), emergency rooms, catheterization laboratories, and surgical suites. However, many of these devices are not suitable for ST monitoring, although the displayed ECG signal may show ST-segment abnormalities. Often, distortions of the low-frequency content of the signal caused by inadequate filtering techniques and "baseline wander correction" may result in distortion of the morphology of the ST segment.[34] Furthermore, in most systems, only one lead is displayed on the central monitoring station, although many systems currently record two or three leads simultaneously. Lead orientation is focused on the detection of arrhythmia rather than ischemia, which results in decreased sensitivity for ST episodes occurring in areas other than the lead monitored.[34-37] Also, fatigue of the medical staff, due partly to the display of tracings from several patients simultaneously, results in under-reporting of ST episodes.[38] Thus, arrhythmia monitoring systems can be used reliably for ST monitoring only if: 1) filtering techniques provide an adequate low-frequency response; 2) lead orientation allows detection of both ischemia and arrhythmias; and 3) proper ischemia detection algorithms are integrated, including storage of complexes and measurements for comparison in full disclosure format and trending of the ST-segment deviation over time.

The major disadvantage of Holter recorders applied in continuous ST monitoring is that retrospective off-line analysis does not allow real-time triage at the bedside. Therefore, Holter ST monitoring should be restricted to use in comparative trials and research.[25,39-41] The number of leads monitored is restricted. A three-lead system with a (pseudo-) orthogonal orientation (such as an anterior lead V_2, apical lead V_5, and an inferior lead aVF or III) should be preferred so that sufficient injury current is recorded for ST-segment recovery analysis.[35-37] It also is important to realize that ST-segment amplitudes measured on the bipolar Holter recordings are not fully comparable with ones measured on the unipolar precordial leads of the 12-lead ECG.[42] An advantage of Holter ST monitoring is that it records all beats without front-end selection or classification, making it appropriate for the parallel analysis of ST-segment recovery and arrhythmias in full disclosure.[43,44] Furthermore, many clinics already have Holter recorders for the purpose of arrhythmia monitoring and, often, the system is also suitable for ST-segment monitoring, with an adequate frequency response and an adequate analysis system. Familiarity with the device and financial considerations will lower the threshold for these hospitals to participate in multicenter trials using ST-monitoring technology.

Continuously Updated ST-Segment Recovery Analysis for Patency Assessment

The general principles of continuously updated ST-segment recovery analysis using continuous 12-lead ST-segment recordings or vector ECG recordings have been described in detail[1,3,4] and are summarized in Figure 4. In patients with acute myocardial infarction, multiple episodes of ST-segment recovery and recurrent elevation, reflecting reperfusion and reocclusion of the infarct-related artery, may occur. Thus, the algorithm focuses on the identification of "troughs" and "peaks" in the trendline of ST-segment deviation over time, representing reperfusion and reocclusion, respectively. Often, a single lead with the most ST-segment elevation is selected, but a trendline of summated ST-segment deviation or ST-vector magnitude may be preferred in the presence of extensive ischemia over multiple leads. During a peak period of ongoing or worsening of ST-segment elevation, the reference ECG is continuously updated to the ECG with the most severe ST-segment elevation. ST-segment recovery of 50% or more from this ECG with the most ST-segment elevation is used to define the onset of a trough representing reperfusion. During such periods of ST-segment recovery, the reference ECG is continuously updated to the ECG with the least ST-segment elevation. Subsequent ST-segment reelevation in the same "fingerprint" pattern (ST-segment deviation over the 12 leads that matches the pattern of the first occlusion episode), requiring 100 μV to 200 μV or more in a single lead relative to the most ST-normalized ECG, is used to define the onset of a new peak episode representing reocclusion. Subsequent points of maximal or minimal ST-segment deviation are used as continuously updated reference points over the entire recording of the ST monitor. Formal quantitative algorithms based on these general principles have been compared with a simultaneous assessment of patency by coronary angiography[1,2,4] (see below).

Early and rapid stabilization of the QRS vector difference may also indicate reperfusion.[3] However, in a study of patients with only minor changes in the ST trend, the benefit from monitoring QRS vector changes in addition to ST-segment changes was marginal.[3]

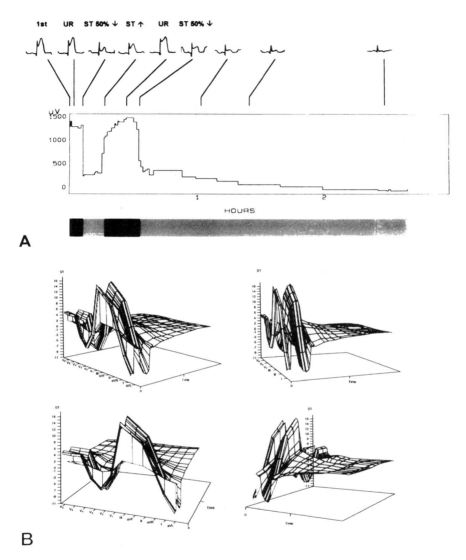

Figure 4. A. The general principles of continuously updated ST-segment recovery analysis using continuous ST-segment recordings are shown. In patients with acute myocardial infarction, multiple episodes of ST-segment recovery and recurrent elevation, reflecting reperfusion and reocclusion of the infarct-related artery, may occur. The algorithm focuses on the identification of "troughs" and "peaks" in the trendline of ST deviation over time, representing reperfusion and reocclusion, respectively. A single lead with the most ST-segment elevation is selected, in this case lead III. The first ECG displays 13-mm ST-segment elevation in lead III. During a peak period of

Accuracy of Patency Assessment

Comparison With
Coronary Angiography

Table 2 lists the performance variables of four studies using continuously updated ST-segment recovery analysis to predict simultaneous angiographic coronary flow status of the infarct-related artery.[1-4] Although the sensitivity to predict reocclusion needs to be improved, continuously updated ST-segment recovery analysis has been shown to be a useful noninvasive indicator of coronary flow status. The accuracy of patency assessment has been shown to be better in patients with higher initial ST-segment elevation than in those with only minimal ST-segment elevation.[4] Most likely, this is because the higher ST-segment amplitudes will result in a better definition of peaks and troughs in the trendline of ST-segment deviation over time. The results of a recent retrospective study suggest that patients with low peak ST-segment amplitudes (≤ 200 μV) have a benign prognosis regardless of the location of the infarction or the perfusion status of the infarct-related artery on early angiography.[45] Thus, the decreased accuracy of ST-monitoring

---

ongoing or worsening ST-segment elevation, the reference ECG is continuously updated to the ECG with the most severe ST-segment elevation. In this recording, the second ECG has increased ST-segment elevation, thus being an updated reference (UR). ST-segment recovery of $\geq 50\%$ from this most ST-segment-elevated ECG is used to define the onset of a trough representing reperfusion. During such periods of ST-segment recovery, the reference ECG is continuously updated to the ECG with the least ST-segment elevation. At this moment, the first ECG with $\geq 50\%$ ST-segment recovery is also the most normalized ECG. Subsequent ST reelevation ≥ 150 μV in the same "fingerprint" pattern (ST deviation over the 12 leads that matches the pattern of the first occlusion episode relative to this most ST-normalized ECG) is used to define the onset of a new peak episode representing reocclusion. Subsequent points of maximal or minimal ST deviation are used as continuously updated reference points over the entire recording of the ST monitor. With this algorithm, two episodes of coronary occlusion (**solid bars at the bottom**) and two episodes of coronary reperfusion (**hatched bars**) are identified. **B.** Three-dimensional displays of ST deviation (Y-axis) in all 12 leads (X-axis) over time (Z-axis) in four spatial rotations of the same ST recording of a patient with acute myocardial infarction, as seen in Figure 4A. A clear representation of each of the axes is seen in the first rotation (**upper left**). The second rotation (**lower left**) clearly shows that the initial ST-segment elevation is most prominent in the inferior leads II, aVF, and III, with additional ST-segment elevation in leads V_4, V_5, and V_6. ST-segment depression occurs in V_2, V_3, I, and aVL. This pattern establishes the "fingerprint-pattern" of ST deviation that disappears with reperfusion through the infarct-related artery and occurs again in the second occlusion episode, although the ST amplitudes are different. The third and fourth rotations show the ST resolution and reelevation over time.

Table 2
Four Studies Reporting Performance of Continuously Updated ST-Segment
Recovery Analysis in Comparison With Simultaneous Coronary Angiography

Author	No. of Observations	TIMI 0–1, *%	Sensitivity, †%	Specificity, ‡%	Accuracy, §%	PPV, ‖%	NPV, ¶%	Comments
Krucoff et al[1]	22	#	90	92	#	#	#	Pilot study, formal algorithm, not blinded, few data on performance
Krucoff et al[2]	144	27	64	90	83	71	87	Correct study design, formal algorithm
Dellborg et al[3]	96	27	73	83	80	61	89	Correct study design, both ST and QRS information used, partially formalized algorithm
Klootwijk et al[4]	302	35	44	84	70	59	74	Complex study design, formal simple algorithm, late onset of monitoring relatively inexperienced participating centers

NPV = negative predictive value; PPV = positive predictive value; TIMI 0–1 = Thrombolysis in Myocardial Infarction flow grade 0 or 1.

* All studies considered TIMI flow grade 2 or 3 to reflect infarct related artery patency, and the presence or absence of collateral blood supply was not taken into account.

† Ability to detect an angiographically occluded infarct-related artery.

‡ Ability to correctly predict an angiographically open infarct-related artery.

§ Percentage of correct predictions overall.

‖ Percentage of correct predictions of an occluded infarct-related artery.

¶ Percentage of correct predictions of a patent infarct-related artery.

Information was not reported or reconstructible from the data given.

(Reproduced with permission from Reference 59.)

patency assessment in patients with low peak ST-segment amplitudes may be tolerable in clinical decision making because, in any event, these patients may have less benefit from secondary reperfusion strategies.

Lowering the threshold for the definition of reocclusion may result in a better sensitivity for detecting reocclusion. Furthermore, the time frame of 1 to 3 hours, in which 50% recovery from the most abnormal ECG defines the onset of a reperfusion episode, may be shortened to better distinguish actual reperfusion-induced ST-segment recovery from loss of ST-segment amplitude due to loss of ischemic myocardial mass (burn-out) in ongoing coronary occlusion.[1,2,4] However, both suggested changes in a prospectively tested formal algorithm may also decrease specificity. A prospective study of the effects of these changes on accuracy, as compared with coronary angiography, should be performed before these changes are implemented.

Use of continuously updated ST-segment recovery analysis has not been validated in patients with delayed ventricular conduction, but they comprise only a small part of the population of patients with acute myocardial infarction.[2,11] More restricting is the requirement that the initial ST-segment deviation indicating coronary occlusion is still present when ST monitoring is initiated. In fact, accuracy of patency assessment by continuous ST-segment recovery analysis strongly depends on peak ST-segment deviation.[4] This requirement favors the analysis of anterior over inferior infarctions and both over posterior infarctions.[37,46] Availability of hard-copy ECGs recorded during coronary occlusion can substitute missing data before ST monitoring is initiated, but this limits the detection of the onset and stability of reperfusion.

Thrombolysis in Myocardial Infarction Investigation Grade 2 Flow and Collateral Blood Supply

In recent studies, thrombolysis in myocardial infarction investigation (TIMI) grade 2 flow has been considered a failure of thrombolytic therapy to achieve complete reperfusion, resulting in unfavorable outcomes in relation to patients with TIMI grade 3 flow.[47,48] It is unfortunate that all four studies mentioned in Table 2 defined TIMI grade 2 flow as "patent"[1-4]; furthermore, collateral blood supply to the infarct area was not taken into consideration in any of these studies. Results of a retrospective analysis of ST-segment recovery analysis versus angiographic flow status in the 144 patients of the ST-monitoring study of the Thrombolysis and Angioplasty in Myocardial Infarction (TAMI)-7 trial are shown in Table 3.[2] Of the 27 patients with TIMI grade 2 flow on early angiography, 5 (19%) had persistent or recurrent ST-segment elevation, suggesting ongoing infarction. In contrast, only 5 (6%) of the 78 patients with TIMI grade 3 flow had ongoing or recurrent ST-segment elevation. Of the patients with collateralized occlusion, 43% had persistent or recurrent ST-segment elevation, suggesting ongoing infarction, in comparison with 89% of the patients with noncollateralized occlusion. These data suggest that ST-segment recovery analysis may result in a better definition of prognosis within these subgroups than angiographic flow assessment alone,[2,49] as discussed below.

Table 3
Results of a Retrospective Analysis of ST-Segment
Recovery Analysis Versus Angiographic Flow Status
in 144 Patients From the TAMI-7 ST-Monitoring
Study

	Ongoing or Recurrent ST-Segment Elevation	
TIMI Flow Grade	No. of Patients	%
3	5/78	6
2	5/27	19
0–1	25/39	64
0–1 with collaterals	9/21	43
0–1 without collaterals	16/18	89

TAMI = Thrombolysis and Angioplasty in Myocardial Infarction; TIMI = Thrombolysis in Myocardial Infarction.
(Data reproduced with permission from Reference 2.)

Comparison of Continuous ST-Segment Recovery Analysis With Static ECG Methods

Several methods using assessment of ST-segment recovery between a single pretreatment ECG and a static post-treatment ECG have been correlated with patency of the infarct-related artery.[28–33] The added demand for a dedicated ST monitor and use of a more complex algorithm for continuously updated ST-segment recovery analysis have been weighed against these simpler static ECG methods in 82 patients with acute myocardial infarction from the TAMI-7 trial with angiography a median of 124 minutes after the onset of thrombolytic treatment.[24] Accuracy (95% confidence limits) at the moment of angiography was 85% (77% to 93%) for the continuous method and 68% (57% to 78%), 78% (69% to 87%), 83% (74% to 91%), 82% (73% to 90%), and 80% (71% to 89%) for the different static methods. At the moment of angiography 2 hours after the onset of thrombolytic therapy, the most accurate static method and the continuous method agreed in patency assessment in 90% of the patients (84% to 97%). Agreement was decreased to 83% (75% to 91%) when a patency assessment was performed 90 minutes after treatment onset and was only 77% (68% to 86%) at 60 minutes. Early disagreement was found mainly when the continuous ST recording showed ST-segment recovery from a delayed peak ST-segment elevation following the pretreatment static ECG or when dynamic ST-segment changes suggested cyclic reperfusion. Thus, continuous ST-segment recovery analysis appeared to give important additional information when ST-segment recovery followed a delayed peak ST-segment elevation or when reelevation occurred, suggesting cyclic flow changes. Such findings occur in about one half of the patients with acute myocardial infarction treated with intravenous thrombolysis, particularly early after initiation of therapy. As illustated in Figure 5, continuously updated ST-segment recovery analysis will result in earlier recognition of reperfusion through the infarct-related artery when ST-segment recovery follows a delayed peak ST-segment elevation. Figure 6 shows ST-segment behavior over time in a patient with multiple ST-segment recovery and reelevation episodes, suggesting intermittent reperfusion through the infarct-related artery. Depending on the moment of acquisition of the static baseline (pretreatment) ECG and on the moment of acquisition of the assessment (post-treatment) ECG, a static ECG method will lead to assessments different from those of continuously updated ST-recovery analysis. Moreover, when only two ECGs are recorded, the presence of intermittent reperfusion will not be recognized. The failure to detect intermittent reperfusion, with its potential adverse effect on prognosis[8,25] (see section on *Physiology*), may lead to a clinical decision that redirects therapy away from treatments designed to maintain an open infarct-related artery (see section on *ST Monitoring for Triage Following Thrombolytic Treatment*).

Comparing and Combining ST Monitoring With Other Patency Assessment Methods

The presence or absence of reperfusion can be detected by rapid assays of myocardial proteins in the plasma, for example, the enzyme creatine kinase and its cardiospecific isoform, myoglobin, and troponin T.[32,50–53] An early increase in the plasma levels of any of these proteins indicates reperfusion. Patency assessments based on differences in the rate of appearance of these myocardial proteins in the plasma between patients with and those without reperfusion should be preferred above determination of the time from treatment to peak plasma levels, because waiting for the peaks to occur with serial plasma determinations delays clinical triage.[40,52] Simple assays that can be performed 24 hours a day, preferably by coronary care unit personnel, and with rapid results, are essential for clinical usefulness.[40,52] Serial enzyme assays may indicate the presence of cyclic reperfusion, as shown in Figure 7.[40] Recurrent occlusion will be detected only when subsequent reperfusion results in a second increase in released enzymes. Application of serial enzyme assays for dynamic patency monitoring requires further development.

Early occurring accelerated idioventricular rhythm (AIVR) seems

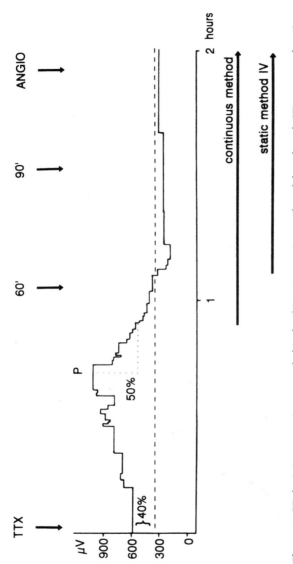

Figure 5. ST deviation over time recorded in lead V₂, in a patient with a delayed peak ST-segment elevation. When the continuous method identified 50% ST-segment recovery from a delayed peak (P) and assessed the infarct artery as patent, the static method[33] predicted an occluded infarct artery, because ST-segment recovery had not yet progressed below the fixed threshold of 40% ST-segment recovery from the pretreatment ECG reference ST level (**dashed line**). Further ST recovery progressed below the static method's threshold 13 minutes later, leading to concordance in assessment from that moment onward. Thus, while the continuous method and static method disagree in patency assessment at 60 minutes after onset of thrombolytic therapy, they agree at 90 minutes and at the moment of angiography, almost 2 hours after onset of treatment. The **four vertical arrows** indicate timing of the following: onset of thrombolytic therapy (TTX), patency assessments performed at 60 minutes (60') and 90 minutes (90') after onset of treatment, and the moment of angiography (ANGIO). The **two horizontal arrows** indicate the time during which the continuous method or static method would assess the infarct-related artery as patent. Angiography revealed TIMI grade 3 flow through a proximal left anterior descending artery lesion. (Reproduced with permission from Reference 24.)

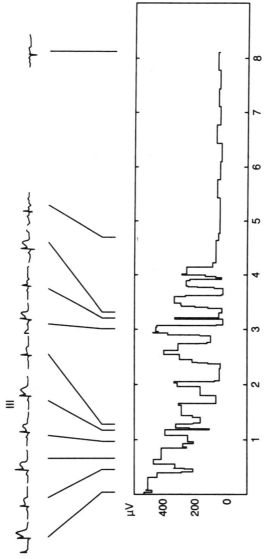

Figure 6. Trend of ST deviation over time recorded in lead III. This tracing shows 11 episodes of recurrent ST-segment elevation, suggesting 11 episodes of reocclusion in the 4 hours after onset of thrombolytic treatment. It is likely that this intermittent reperfusion pattern was also present before onset of thrombolytic treatment. Depending on the moment of acquisition of the baseline ECG and on the moment of acquisition of the post-treatment assessment ECG, a static patency-predicting method will lead to a different, possibly erroneous assessment of patency. Moreover, when only two ECGs are recorded, the presence of intermittent reperfusion will not be recognized.

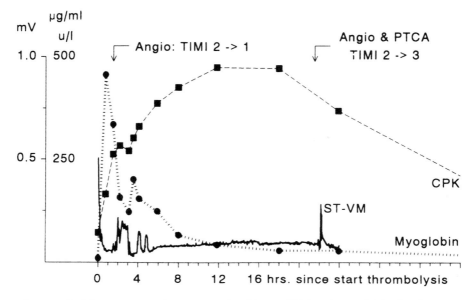

Figure 7. Serial assessment of serum creatine kinase (CPK) and myoglobin simultaneously with continuous vectorcardiographic registration of the ST-segment vector magnitude (ST-VM). The early increase in myoglobin is more rapid than that of CPK and both coincide with rapid ST-VM recovery. A second small increase in myoglobin paralleled reelevation of the ST-segment, secondary to reocclusion of the infarct-related artery. Angio = angiography; PTCA = percutaneously transluminal coronary angioplasty; TIMI = Thrombolysis in Myocardial Infarction Flow grade. (Reproduced with permission from Reference 40.)

to be the most reliable of the "reperfusion arrhythmias."[32,54–58] The combined analysis of six studies (317 patients) reporting on the accuracy of patency assessment with early AIVR supports the assumption that it predicts reperfusion with high specificity (97%) but low sensitivity (45%), because of its infrequent incidence of 35%.[59] However, a direct temporal relationship between ST-segment recovery as a marker of reperfusion and the occurrence of reperfusion arrhythmias was not found in one study.[43] Moreover, AIVR cannot indicate reocclusion.

As mentioned above, ST monitoring is not applicable in two situations. First, it has not been validated in patients with delayed ventricular conduction, but these patients comprise a small part of the population with acute myocardial infarction.[2,11] More restricting is the requirement that the initial ST-segment deviation reflecting coronary occlusion should be present when ST monitoring is initiated. The accuracy of patency assessment with continuous ST-segment recovery analysis strongly depends on monitored peak ST-segment deviation.[4] When

ST monitoring is not applicable, either biochemical assays or arrhythmia monitoring is a logical alternative. The integration of AIVR detection algorithms into an ST-monitoring environment seems logical. Parallel application of ST monitoring, with a two-point biochemical assay or arrhythmia monitoring (or both) might increase the accuracy of predicting patency,[32] and it would provide a backup assessment in case of failure of one of the methods.[39] However, more studies are needed to understand fully the relationship among these three indicators of reperfusion.

Applications of ST Monitoring During Myocardial Infarction

ST Monitoring for Triage Following Thrombolytic Treatment

To avoid unnecessary bleeding risk,[60] thrombolytic therapy might be discontinued in patients with acute myocardial infarction when ST-segment recovery indicates early reperfusion of the infarct-related artery.[61,62] Patients with acute myocardial infarction in whom thrombolytic therapy fails to provide early and stable reperfusion might benefit from additional treatment, such as rescue angioplasty, rescue thrombolysis, or from additional medical treatment, such as antithrombin or antiplatelet compounds.[21,63–73] Figure 8 illustrates the possible treatment options that could be chosen depending on the reperfusion behavior, as indicated by continuously updated ST-segment recovery analysis. Many of these options are being debated or have not been investigated, partly because a useful (continuous) noninvasive patency assessment method was not available until the development of continuous real-time ECG analysis. These options include discontinuing thrombolytic treatment after reperfusion has been achieved, rescue thrombolytic therapy, and rescue coronary angioplasty. Further research on the reperfusion patterns following thrombolytic therapy and treatment strategies dependent on the specific reperfusion pattern is required so that treatment regimens can be optimized according to a patient's response.

ST Monitoring in Clinical Trials

Because mortality after acute myocardial infarction is relatively infrequent, studies with a mortality end point require large study populations. Thus, infarct size, left ventricular function, and angiographic patency of the infarct-related artery have been used as alternative end points to compare treatment strategies. Because angiography is not available in every hospital, there is increased interest in simple nonin-

ST pattern	Suggesting	Clinical	Suggested action
	Early stable reperfusion	Small infarct size electrical stability Survival ↑	Stop thrombolytic therapy
	Early cyclic reperfusion	Large infarct size Survival ↓	Stop thrombolytic therapy Anti-coagulants Platelet inhibitors Vasodilators ↑
	No reperfusion	Large infarct size electrical stability Survival ↓↑	Repeat thrombolytic therapy Urgent angiography & PTCA
	Late recurrent occlusion	Recurrent infarction Survival ↓↑	Repeat thrombolytic therapy Urgent angiography & PTCA

vasive patency assessments.[82,83] Early opening of the infarct-related artery is related directly to limitation of infarct size, preservation of left ventricular function, and better clinical outcome.[47,48,74−78] Previous studies have shown the unfavorable results of reocclusion.[8,25,79,80] The documentation and timing of reperfusion and the assessment of reocclusion with continuously updated ST-segment recovery analysis might be important surrogate end points in trials comparing drug regimens aimed at early stable reperfusion for the improvement of prognosis after acute myocardial infarction.[39,49,82,83]

ST Monitoring to Determine Prognosis

Besides the possibility of tailoring thrombolytic and adjuvant therapy to a patient's individual response, continuous real-time ST monitoring might be helpful in determining the prognosis of a patient. Barbash and coworkers[84] showed in a series of 286 patients that a decrease in the summated ST-segment elevation of 50% or more from the admission ECG 1 hour after the onset of treatment with alteplase (rTPA) was associated with a significantly smaller infarct size (release of creatine kinase), better preservation of left ventricular function, lower morbidity, and

◄─────────────────────────────────────

Figure 8. Possible treatment options (**right column**) that could be chosen depending on the reperfusion behavior following thrombolytic therapy for acute myocardial infarction as evidenced by continuously updated 12-lead ST-segment recovery analysis (**two columns on the left side**). In the three-dimensional graphs in the far left column, the X-axis represents each of the 12 leads, the Y-axis represents the ST deviation measured 60 ms after J-point, and the Z-axis represents time.[1] The **third column** explains the clinical implications of the different types of reperfusion behavior. Early stable reperfusion is associated with limitations of infarct size, electrical stability of the myocardium, and improved survival.[47,48,74−79] Early cyclic reperfusion is associated with large infarct size and decreased survival.[8,25] No reperfusion is related to larger infarcts, electrical instability, and decreased survival.[47,48,74−78] Reocclusion, potentially resulting in recurrent infarction, is associated with increased morbidity and mortality.[8,25,79−81] It has been suggested that thrombolytic therapy may be stopped after ST-segment recovery, signifying reperfusion has occurred.[60−62] When ST recovery is followed by recurrent ST-segment elevation, suggesting cyclic reperfusion, the addition of anticoagulants, platelet inhibitors, or higher doses of vasodilators may be helpful in stabilizing reperfusion.[21,63−66] When no reperfusion occurs following thrombolytic therapy or when late reocclusion occurs, rescue thrombolytic therapy[67−69] or angiography with rescue percutaneous transluminal coronary angioplasty (PTCA)[70−72] or intracoronary thrombolytic therapy[73] may be considered. Trials testing these strategies after triage with continuously updated ST-segment recovery analysis and other noninvasive patency assessments are warranted. (Reproduced with permission from Reference 59.)

Table 4

Relation Between Rapid ST-Segment Recovery After Treatment With Recombinant Tissue Plasminogen Activator*

	Rapid ST-Segment Recovery		
Variable	Yes (n = 189)	No (n = 97)	P
24-hr total CK release†	5,248 IU (SD, 4,265)	10,553 IU (SD, 7,762)	<0.001
LVEF at dismissal‡	55% (SD, 12)	44% (SD, 14)	<0.001
60-day mortality	3 (1.6%)	10 (10.3%)	0.0015
CHF during hospitalization§	8 (4.2%)	18 (18.6%)	<0.001

CHF = congestive heart failure; CK = creatine kinase; LVEF = left ventricular ejection fraction; SD = standard deviation.

* ≥50% reduction in summated ST deviation within 1 hour after treatment onset.

† Area under the curve of several samples.

‡ Assessed with radionuclide-gated blood pool scan.

§ CHF at admission excluded patients for this study.

(Data reproduced with permission from Reference 84.)

improved short- and long-term survival (Table 4 and Figure 9). It is noteworthy that the summated ST-segment elevation at admission had no independent predictive value for clinical outcome when the presence or absence of ST-segment recovery was taken into account. Saran and coworkers[30] also found that rapid ST-segment recovery was associated with preservation of left ventricular function.

Schröder and coworkers,[49] from the Internal Joint Efficacy Comparison of Thrombolytics (INJECT) trial, prospectively assessed the prognostic power of early resolution of ST-segment elevation in 1,398 patients presenting 6 hours or less after the onset of acute myocardial infarction. Three groups of patients were defined according to an ECG performed 3 hours after onset of thrombolytic treatment (range, 2 to 4 hours): complete ST-segment resolution (≥ 70%); partial resolution (69% to 30%); or no resolution (< 30%) of the initial summated ST-segment elevation, as seen in the pretreatment ECG. The 35-day mortality and peak creatine kinase levels in each of these three groups are summarized in Table 5. When baseline characteristics were included, ST-segment resolution was the most powerful predictor of 35-day mortality.

Preliminary data from a study using continuous ST monitoring showed that patients without ST-segment reelevation (indicating lack

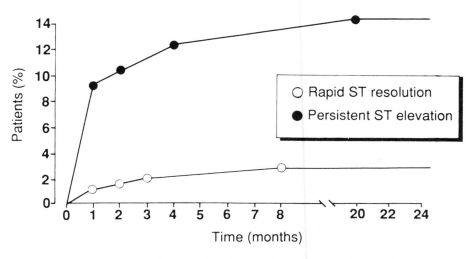

Figure 9. Cumulative mortality (%) of patients with rapid resolution of ST-segment elevation and those without. (Reprodcued with permission from Reference 84.)

Table 5
Relation Between Amount of ST-Segment Recovery 3 Hours* After Treatment With Intravenous Reteplase or Streptokinase and 35-Day Mortality and Peak Creatine Kinase Level as Seen in the INJECT Trial

ST-Segment Resolution 3 Hours After Treatment Onset	Mortality		Peak Creatine Kinase Level,† as Fraction of Normal
	No. of Patients	%	
Complete (≥70%)	17/682	2.5	9.8
Partial (69% to 30%)	18/418	4.3	13.4
None (<30%)	52/298	17	14.0

* Range, 2 to 4 hours.
† Differences in mortality and peak creatine kinase per ST-recovery group were statistically significant ($P < 0.0001$).
(Data reproduced with permission from Reference 49.)

of reocclusion more than 3 hours after the onset of thrombolytic therapy) have a lower morbidity and mortality than patients with unstable or failed reperfusion after 3 hours.[81]

The prognostic importance of variables derived from continuous monitoring, such as the presence and timing of rapid ST-segment recovery, maximum amplitude and extent of the infarct zone, time to reperfusion, and early or late stability of reperfusion, needs to be explored in large groups of patients. Prognostic ST-segment recovery variables should be compared and combined with other noninvasive clinical information (e.g., age, history of angina, history of previous infarction, treatment delay, reperfusion therapy administered, infarct size, left ventricular function, and presence of congestive heart failure).[47] Clinical models may be developed so that risk stratification and, thus, medical care after reperfusion therapy can be individualized. Ideally, the duration of the hospital stay can be shortened or lengthened on the basis of individual risk assessments. For example, a very low risk of complications could lead to a shorter stay in the coronary care unit, followed by earlier release.[85,86] However, patients at high risk would require a longer period of observation in the coronary care unit. Models predicting long-term prognosis could also include outcomes of early ambulatory ST monitoring after release from the coronary care unit[87,88] or exercise treadmill ECG before or after hospital release.[89-91]

Conclusion

Continuously updated ST-segment recovery analysis is a useful noninvasive patency assessment technique that allows, with reasonable accuracy, the identification of failed or unstable reperfusion and reocclusion after thrombolytic therapy for acute myocardial infarction. Automated multilead ECG devices with real-time accessibility of recorded ECGs are preferred and are commercially available. This technique can be used to select patients for rescue strategies in case of failed or unstable reperfusion or reocclusion or for discontinuation of thrombolytic therapy after reperfusion has occurred.

Continuously updated ST-segment recovery analysis as an end point in acute myocardial infarction trials comparing treatment strategies aimed at early stable reperfusion of the infarct-related artery deserves exploration as an additional end point beyond a snapshot patency assessment with coronary angiography.

Although more studies on the prognostic value of ST monitoring-derived variables of presence and stability of reperfusion are required, it has been shown that the presence of early and stable ST-segment resolution as an indicator of reperfusion defines a subgroup of patients with small infarcts and excellent prognosis. These patients may be suitable candidates for early discharge after acute myocardial infarction.

References

1. Krucoff MW, Croll MA, Pope JE, et al: Continuously updated 12-lead ST-segment recovery analysis for myocardial infarct artery patency assessment and its correlation with multiple simultaneous early angiographic observations. *Am J Cardiol* 71:145–151, 1993.
2. Krucoff MW, Croll MA, Pope JE, et al: Continuous 12-lead ST-segment recovery analysis in the TAMI 7 study. Performance of a noninvasive method for real-time detection of failed myocardial reperfusion. *Circulation* 88:437–446, 1993.
3. Dellborg M, Steg PG, Simoons M, et al: Vectorcardiographic monitoring to assess early vessel patency after reperfusion therapy for acute myocardial infarction. *Eur Heart J* 16:21–29, 1995.
4. Klootwijk P, Langer A, Meij S, et al: Non-invasive prediction of reperfusion and coronary artery patency by continuous ST segment monitoring in the GUSTO-I trial. *Eur Heart J* 17:689–698, 1996.
5. von Essen R, Hinsen R, Louis R, et al: On-line monitoring of multiple precordial leads in high risk patients with coronary artery disease—a pilot study. *Eur Heart J* 5:203–209, 1984.
6. Sederholm M: Monitoring of acute myocardial infarct evolution by continuous spatial electrocardiography. In: Califf RM, Mark DB, Wagner GS (eds): *Acute Coronary Care in the Thrombolytic Era*. Chicago: Year Book Medical Publishers; 444–458, 1988.
7. Dellborg M, Riha M, Swedberg K: Dynamic QRS and ST-segment changes in myocardial infarction monitored by continuous on-line vectorcardiography. *J Electrocardiol* 23(suppl):11–19, 1990.
8. Dellborg M, Riha M, Swedberg K: Dynamic QRS-complex and ST-segment monitoring in acute myocardial infarction during recombinant tissue-type plasminogen activator therapy. *Am J Cardiol* 67:343–349, 1991.
9. Adams IM, Mortara DW: A new method for electrocardiographic monitoring. In: Califf RM, Wagner GS (eds): *Acute Coronary Care 1987*. Boston: Martinus Nijhoff; 165–176, 1987.
10. Krucoff MW, Wagner NB, Pope JE, et al: The portable programmable microprocessor-driven real-time 12-lead electrocardiographic monitor: a preliminary report of a new device for the noninvasive detection of successful reperfusion or silent coronary reocclusion. *Am J Cardiol* 65:143–148, 1990.
11. Rude RE, Poole WK, Muller JE, et al: Electrocardiographic and clinical criteria for recognition of acute myocardial infarction based on analysis of 3,697 patients. *Am J Cardiol* 52:936–942, 1983.
12. Thygesen K, Hörder M, Nielsen BL, Petersen PH: The variability of ST segment in the early phase of acute myocardial infarction. *Acta Med Scand Suppl* 623:61–70, 1978.
13. Yusuf S, Pearson M, Sterry H, et al: The entry ECG in the early diagnosis and prognostic stratification of patients with suspected acute myocardial infarction. *Eur Heart J* 5:690–696, 1984.
14. Yusuf S, Lopez R, Maddison A, et al: Value of electrocardiogram in predicting and estimating infarct size in man. *Br Heart J* 42:286–293, 1979.
15. Bar FW, Vermeer F, de Zwaan C, et al: Value of admission electrocardiogram in predicting outcome of thrombolytic therapy in acute myocardial infarction. A randomized trial conducted by The Netherlands Interuniversity Cardiology Institute. *Am J Cardiol* 59:6–13, 1987.

16. Aldrich HR, Wagner NB, Boswick J, et al: Use of initial ST-segment deviation for prediction of final electrocardiographic size of acute myocardial infarcts. *Am J Cardiol* 61:749–753, 1988.
17. Willems JL, Willems RJ, Willems GM, Arnold AE, Van de Werf F, Verstraete M: Significance of initial ST segment elevation and depression for the management of thrombolytic therapy in acute myocardial infarction. *Circulation* 82: 1147–1158, 1990.
18. Anderson JL, Marshall HW, Bray BE, et al: A randomized trial of intracoronary streptokinase in the treatment of acute myocardial infarction. *N Engl J Med* 308: 1312–1318, 1983.
19. Blanke H, Scherff F, Karsch KR, Levine RA, Smith H, Rentrop P: Electrocardiographic changes after streptokinase-induced recanalization in patients with acute left anterior descending artery obstruction. *Circulation* 68:406–412, 1983.
20. Krucoff MW, Green CE, Satler LF, et al: Noninvasive detection of coronary artery patency using continuous ST-segment monitoring. *Am J Cardiol* 57:916–922, 1986.
21. Hackett D, Davies G, Chierchia S, Maseri A: Intermittent coronary occlusion in acute myocardial infarction. Value of combined thrombolytic and vasodilator therapy. *N Engl J Med* 317:1055–1059, 1987.
22. Davies GJ, Chierchia S, Maseri A: Prevention of myocardial infarction by very early treatment with intracoronary streptokinase. Some clinical observations. *N Engl J Med* 311:1488–1492, 1984.
23. Kwon K, Freedman SB, Wilcox I, et al: The unstable ST segment early after thrombolysis for acute infarction and its usefulness as a marker of recurrent coronary occlusion. *Am J Cardiol* 67:109–115, 1991.
24. Veldkamp RF, Green CL, Wilkins ML, et al: Comparison of continuous ST-segment recovery analysis with methods using static electrocardiograms for noninvasive patency assessment during acute myocardial infarction. *Am J Cardiol* 73: 1069–1074, 1994.
25. Langer A, Krucoff MW, Klootwijk P, et al: Noninvasive assessment of speed and stability of infarct-related artery reperfusion: results of the GUSTO ST segment monitoring study. *J Am Coll Cardiol* 25:1552–1557, 1995.
26. Maseri A, Chierchia S, Davies G: Pathophysiology of coronary occlusion in acute infarction. *Circulation* 73:233–239, 1986.
27. Cohen M, Rentrop KP: Limitation of myocardial ischemia by collateral circulation during sudden controlled coronary artery occlusion in human subjects: a prospective study. *Circulation* 74:469–476, 1986.
28. von Essen R, Schmidt W, Uebis R, et al: Myocardial infarction and thrombolysis. Electrocardiographic short-term and long-term results using precordial mapping. *Br Heart J* 54:6–10, 1985.
29. Hogg KJ, Hornung RS, Howie CA, Hockings N, Dunn FG, Hillis WS: Electrocardiographic prediction of coronary artery patency after thrombolytic treatment in acute myocardial infarction: use of the ST segment as a non-invasive marker. *Br Heart J* 60:275–280, 1988.
30. Saran RK, Been M, Furniss SS, Hawkins T, Reid DS: Reduction in ST segment elevation after thrombolysis predicts either coronary reperfusion or preservation of left ventricular function. *Br Heart J* 64:113–117, 1990.
31. Clemmensen P, Ohman EM, Sevilla DC, et al: Changes in standard electrocardiographic ST-segment elevation predictive of successful reperfusion in acute myocardial infarction. *Am J Cardiol* 66:1407–1411, 1990.

32. Hohnloser SH, Zabel M, Kasper W, Meinertz T, Just H: Assessment of coronary artery patency after thrombolytic therapy: accurate prediction utilizing the combined analysis of three noninvasive markers. *J Am Coll Cardiol* 18:44–49, 1991.
33. Hackworthy RA, Vogel MB, Harris PJ: Relationship between changes in ST segment elevation and patency of the infarct-related coronary artery in acute myocardial infarction. *Am Heart J* 112:279–284, 1986.
34. Mirvis DM, Berson AS, Goldberger AL, et al: Instrumentation and practice standards for electrocardiographic monitoring in special care units. A report for health professionals by a Task Force of the Council on Clinical Cardiology, American Heart Association. *Circulation* 79:464–471, 1989.
35. Waugh RA, Bride WM, English MB, Wagner GS: The use of electrocardiographic monitoring for diagnosis of cardiac arrhythmias. In: Wagner GS, Waugh RA, Ramo BW (eds): *Cardiac Arrhythmias.* New York: Churchill Livingstone; 108–124, 1983.
36. Aldrich HR, Hindman NB, Hinohara T, et al: Identification of the optimal electrocardiographic leads for detecting acute epicardial injury in acute myocardial infarction. *Am J Cardiol* 59:20–23, 1987.
37. Veldkamp RF, Pope JE, Wilderman NM, et al: ST-segment deviation on the 12-lead electrocardiogram during acute myocardial infarction: optimal leads for continuous ST-segment monitoring. In: Veldkamp RF (ed): *Continuous Digital 12-Lead ST-Segment Monitoring in Acute Myocardial Infarction.* Thesis, Delft, Eburon; 54–66, 1995.
38. Biagini A, L'Abbate A, Testa R, et al: Unreliability of conventional visual electrocardiographic monitoring for detection of transient ST segment changes in a coronary care unit. *Eur Heart J* 5:784–791, 1984.
39. Veldkamp RF, Pope JE, Sawchak ST, Wagner GS, Califf RM, Krucoff MW: ST-segment recovery as an endpoint in acute myocardial infarction trials. Past, present, and future. *J Electrocardiol* 26 (suppl):256–261, 1993.
40. Klootwijk P, Cobbaert C, Fioretti P, Kint PP, Simoons ML: Noninvasive assessment of reperfusion and reocclusion after thrombolysis in acute myocardial infarction. *Am J Cardiol* 72:75G-84G, 1993.
41. Krucoff MW, Green CL, Langer A, et al: Global Utilization of Streptokinase and tPA for Occluded Arteries (GUSTO) ECG-monitoring substudy. Study design and technical considerations. *J Electrocardiol* 26(suppl):249–255, 1993.
42. Krucoff MW, Crater SW, Green CL, et al: Simultaneous Holter, VCG, and ECG ST-monitoring during transient occlusion and reperfusion: implications for comparing or combining data sets (abstr). *Circulation* 88(suppl 1):I-306, 1993.
43. Hackett D, McKenna W, Davies G, Maseri A: Reperfusion arrhythmias are rare during acute myocardial infarction and thrombolysis in man. *Int J Cardiol* 29:205–213, 1990.
44. Gressin V, Gorgels A, Louvard Y, Maison-Blanche P: Reconsidering arrhythmias as markers of reperfusion. Combined arrhythmia and ST-segment analysis during myocardial infarction. *J Electrocardiol* 26(suppl):262–269, 1993.
45. Boineau RE, Green CL, Trollinger KM, Pope JE, Krucoff MW: Interventions may not be necessary in acute myocardial infarction (MI) patients with ≤ 200 μV ST-segment elevation, irrespective of infarct artery patency (abstr). *Circulation* 92(suppl 1):I-740, 1995.
46. Veldkamp RF, Sawchak S, Pope JE, Califf RM, Krucoff MW: Performance of an automated real-time ST-segment analysis program to detect coronary occlusion and reperfusion. *J Electrocardiol* 29:257–263, 1996.

47. Lenderink T, Simoons ML, Van Es GA, Van de Werf F, Verstraete M, Arnold AE: Benefit of thrombolytic therapy is sustained throughout five years and is related to TIMI perfusion grade 3 but not grade 2 flow at discharge. *Circulation* 92: 1110–1116, 1995.

48. Lincoff AM, Topol EJ, Califf RM, et al: Significance of a coronary artery with thrombolysis in myocardial infarction grade 2 flow "patency" (outcome in the Thrombolysis and Angioplasty in Myocardial Infarction Trials). *Am J Cardiol* 75: 871–876, 1995.

49. Schröder R, Wegscheider K, Schroder K, Dissmann R, Meyer-Sabellek W: Extent of early ST segment elevation resolution: a strong predictor of outcome in patients with acute myocardial infarction and a sensitive measure to compare thrombolytic regimens. A substudy of the Internal Joint Efficacy Comparison of Thrombolytics (INJECT) trial. *J Am Coll Cardiol* 26:1657–1664, 1995.

50. Lewis BS, Ganz W, Laramee P, et al: Usefulness of a rapid initial increase in plasma creatine kinase activity as a marker of reperfusion during thrombolytic therapy for acute myocardial infarction. *Am J Cardiol* 62:20–24, 1988.

51. Katus HA, Diederich KW, Scheffold T, Uellner M, Schwarz F, Kubler W: Noninvasive assessment of infarct reperfusion: the predictive power of the time to peak value of myoglobin, CKMB, and CK in serum. *Eur Heart J* 9:619–624, 1988.

52. Zabel M, Hohnloser SH, Koster W, Prinz M, Kasper W, Just H: Analysis of creatine kinase, CK-MB, myoglobin, and troponin T time-activity curves for early assessment of coronary artery reperfusion after intravenous thrombolysis. *Circulation* 87:1542–1550, 1993.

53. Miyata M, Abe S, Arima S, et al: Rapid diagnosis of coronary reperfusion by measurement of myoglobin level every 15 min in acute myocardial infarction. *J Am Coll Cardiol* 23:1009–1015, 1994.

54. Goldberg S, Greenspon AJ, Urban PL, et al: Reperfusion arrhythmia: a marker of restoration of antegrade flow during intracoronary thrombolysis for acute myocardial infarction. *Am Heart J* 105:26–32, 1983.

55. Miller FC, Krucoff MW, Satler LF, et al: Ventricular arrhythmias during reperfusion. *Am Heart J* 112:928–932, 1986.

56. Gorgels AP, Vos MA, Letsch IS, et al: Usefulness of the accelerated idioventricular rhythm as a marker for myocardial necrosis and reperfusion during thrombolytic therapy in acute myocardial infarction. *Am J Cardiol* 61:231–235, 1988.

57. Gore JM, Ball SP, Corrao JM, Goldberg RJ: Arrhythmias in the assessment of coronary artery reperfusion following thrombolytic therapy. *Chest* 94:727–730, 1988.

58. Gressin V, Louvard Y, Pezzano M, Lardoux H: Holter recording of ventricular arrhythmias during intravenous thrombolysis for acute myocardial infarction. *Am J Cardiol* 69:152–159, 1992.

59. Veldkamp RF: *Continuous Digital 12-Lead ST-Segment Monitoring in Acute Myocardial Infarction.* Thesis, Delft, Eburon; 106–111, 1995.

60. Arnold AE, Brower RW, Collen D, et al: Increased serum levels of fibrinogen degradation products due to treatment with recombinant tissue-type plasminogen activator for acute myocardial infarction are related to bleeding complications, but not to coronary patency. *J Am Coll Cardiol* 14:581–588, 1989.

61. Arnold AER, van der Vlugt MJ, Boersma H, Barrett MJ, Burgersdijk C, Simoons ML: Tailored thrombolytic therapy for evolving myocardial infarction: stopping alteplase infusion on signs of reperfusion (abstr). *Eur Heart J* 16(suppl):11, 1995.

62. Simoons ML, Arnold AE: Tailored thrombolytic therapy. A perspective. *Circulation* 88:2556–2564, 1993.
63. Arnout J, Simoons M, de Bono D, Rapold HJ, Collen D, Verstraete M: Correlation between level of heparinization and patency of the infarct-related coronary artery after treatment of acute myocardial infarction with alteplase (rt-PA). *J Am Coll Cardiol* 20:513–519, 1992.
64. The Global Use of Strategies to Open Occluded Coronary Arteries (GUSTO) Ia Investigators: Randomized trial of intravenous heparin versus recombinant hirudin for acute coronary syndromes. *Circulation* 90:1631–1637, 1994.
65. Yao SK, Ober JC, Ferguson JJ, et al: Clopidogrel is more effective than aspirin as adjuvant treatment to prevent reocclusion after thrombolysis. *Am J Physiol* 267:H488-H493, 1994.
66. Kleiman NS, Ohman EM, Califf RM, et al: Profound inhibition of platelet aggregation with monoclonal antibody 7E3 Fab after thrombolytic therapy. Results of the Thrombolysis and Angioplasty in Myocardial Infarction (TAMI) 8 Pilot Study. *J Am Coll Cardiol* 22:381–389, 1993.
67. Barbash GI, Hod H, Roth A, et al: Repeat infusion of recombinant tissue-type plasminogen activator in patients with acute myocardial infarction and early recurrent myocardial ischemia. *J Am Coll Cardiol* 16:779–783, 1990.
68. White HD, Cross DB, Williams BF, Norris RM: Safety and efficacy of repeat thrombolytic treatment after acute myocardial infarction. *Br Heart J* 64:177–181, 1990.
69. Simoons ML, Arnout J, van den Brand M, Nyssen K, Verstraete M: Retreatment with alteplase for early signs of reocclusion after thrombolysis. *Am J Cardiol* 71: 524–528, 1993.
70. Belenkie I, Traboulsi M, Hall CA, et al: Rescue angioplasty during myocardial infarction has a beneficial effect on mortality: a tenable hypothesis. *Can J Cardiol* 8:357–362, 1992.
71. Ellis SG, da Silva ER, Heyndrickx G, et al: Randomized comparison of rescue angioplasty with conservative management of patients with early failure of thrombolysis for acute anterior myocardial infarction. *Circulation* 90: 2280–2284, 1994.
72. Ellis SG, Van de Werf F, Ribeiro-daSilva E, Topol EJ: Present status of rescue coronary angioplasty: current polarization of opinion and randomized trials (editorial). *J Am Coll Cardiol* 19:681–686, 1992.
73. Gurbel PA, Davidson CJ, Ohman EM, Smith JE, Stack RS: Selective infusion of thrombolytic therapy in the acute myocardial infarct-related coronary artery as an alternative to rescue percutaneous transluminal coronary angioplasty. *Am J Cardiol* 66:1021–1023, 1990.
74. Christian TF, Schwartz RS, Gibbons RJ: Determinants of infarct size in reperfusion therapy for acute myocardial infarction. *Circulation* 86:81–90, 1992.
75. The GUSTO Angiographic Investigators: The effects of tissue plasminogen activator, streptokinase, or both on coronary-artery patency, ventricular function, and survival after acute myocardial infarction. *N Engl J Med* 329:1615–1622, 1993.
76. White HD, Cross DB, Elliott JM, Norris RM, Yee TW: Long-term prognostic importance of patency of the infarct-related coronary artery after thrombolytic therapy for acute myocardial infarction. *Circulation* 89:61–67, 1994.
77. Sheehan FH, Mathey DG, Schofer J, Dodge HT, Bolson EL: Factors that determine recovery of left ventricular function after thrombolysis in patients with acute myocardial infarction. *Circulation* 71:1121–1128, 1985.

78. Hohnloser SH, Franck P, Klingenheben T, Zabel M, Just H: Open infarct artery, late potentials, and other prognostic factors in patients after acute myocardial infarction in the thrombolytic era. A prospective trial. *Circulation* 90:1747–1756, 1994.

79. Ohman EM, Califf RM, Topol EJ, et al: Consequences of reocclusion after successful reperfusion therapy in acute myocardial infarction. *Circulation* 82:781–791, 1990.

80. Meijer A, Verheugt FW, van Eenige MJ, Werter CJ: Left ventricular function at 3 months after successful thrombolysis. Impact of reocclusion without reinfarction on ejection fraction, regional function, and remodeling. *Circulation* 90: 1706–1714, 1994.

81. Krucoff MW, Trolinger KM, Veldkamp RF, et al: Detection of recurrent ischemia with continuous electrocardiographic monitoring: early risk stratification following thrombolytic therapy (abstr). *Circulation* 86(suppl 1):I-136, 1992.

82. Editorial: Surrogate measures in clinical trials. *Lancet* 335:261–262, 1990.

83. Hillis WS, Hogg KJ: ST segment changes as a surrogate end point in coronary thrombolysis. *Br Heart J* 64:111–112, 1990.

84. Barbash GI, Roth A, Hod H, et al: Rapid resolution of ST elevation and prediction of clinical outcome in patients undergoing thrombolysis with alteplase (recombinant tissue-type plasminogen activator): results of the Israeli Study of Early Intervention in Myocardial Infarction. *Br Heart J* 64:241–247, 1990.

85. Topol EJ, Burek K, O'Neill WW, et al: A randomized controlled trial of hospital discharge three days after myocardial infarction in the era of reperfusion. *N Engl J Med* 318:1083–1088, 1988.

86. Mark DB, Sigmon K, Topol EJ, et al: Identification of acute myocardial infarction patients suitable for early hospital discharge after aggressive interventional therapy. Results from the Thrombolysis and Angioplasty in Acute Myocardial Infarction Registry. *Circulation* 83:1186–1193, 1991.

87. Gottlieb SO, Gottlieb SH, Achuff SC, et al: Silent ischemia on Holter monitoring predicts mortality in high-risk postinfarction patients. JAMA 259:1030–1035, 1988.

88. Stevenson R, Ranjadayalan K, Wilkinson P, Marchant B, Timmis AD: Assessment of Holter ST monitoring for risk stratification in patients with acute myocardial infarction treated by thrombolysis. *Br Heart J* 70:233–240, 1993.

89. Markiewicz W, Houston N, DeBusk RF: Exercise testing soon after myocardial infarction. Circulation 56:26–31, 1977.

90. Théroux P, Waters DD, Halphen C, Debaisieux JC, Mizgala HF: Prognostic value of exercise testing soon after myocardial infarction. *N Engl J Med* 301:341–345, 1979.

91. Arnold AE, Simoons ML, Detry JM, et al: Prediction of mortality following hospital discharge after thrombolysis for acute myocardial infarction: is there a need for coronary angiography? *Eur Heart J* 14:306–315, 1993.

2

Vectorcardiography in Acute Myocardial Infarction

Ian P. Clements, MD

Introduction

Frank leads, which consist of seven electrodes connected with a number of resistors, allow surface electrocardiograms (ECGs) to be recorded in the three orthogonal planes: frontal, sagittal, and horizontal. The data can be displayed in a scalar manner as the X, Y, and Z leads of the Frank ECG or as three vector loops that trace at each instant the maximal electrical potential and its direction in each of the three orthogonal planes. Both of these display modalities have been used to quantitatively study acute myocardial infarction. Vectorcardiographic methods have advantages over scalar methods. Fewer electrodes are required and their positioning is easier; therefore, the electrodes are less likely to interfere with imaging methods. However, physicians are less familiar with vectorcardiography. Vectorcardiographic recording has been adapted for use in the intensive care setting.[1]

X, Y, and Z Leads and Measurement of Infarct Size

Wikswo and colleagues[2] recorded the X, Y, and Z leads of patients with acute myocardial infarction and proposed a subtraction technique between ECGs obtained at different time intervals after infarction as a

From: Clements, IP (ed). *The Electrocardiogram in Acute Myocardial Infarction.* Armonk, NY: Futura Publishing Company, Inc. © Mayo Foundation 1998.

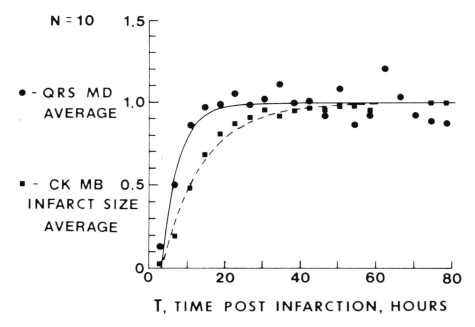

Figure 1. Time course of normalized mean QRS-magnitude difference QRS_{MD} and creatine kinase (CK-MB) data obtained from 10 patients during acute myocardial infarction. (Reproduced with permission from Reference 2.)

means of quantifying infarction. These authors measured the area bounded by the QRS curve in each of the three planes at hourly intervals. The initial QRS area was used as baseline, and the differences between the initial QRS area and the subsequent QRS area were measured at hourly intervals. These values in all three planes at each time interval were summated mathematically and yielded the variable "QRS_{MD}," the magnitude of the difference of the QRS vector in all three planes. Furthermore, the authors established that this variable increased rapidly to a plateau at about 15 hours after infarction, which preceded by a few hours the plateau in release of myocardial creatine kinase (CK-MB) from the infarct zone (Figure 1). The QRS_{MD} had an exponential relationship to time after infarction

$$QRS_{MD}(t) = \alpha \{1 - \alpha^{-\beta(t-to)}\}$$

where t is the time of each measurement and α and β are constants. These constants did not predict final infarct size based on CK-MB release.

Sederholm and coworkers[3] also measured the QRS-vector difference (QRS-VD) (similar to the vector variable described by Wikswo et
al[2]) in patients with acute infarction. The authors also measured the
spatial ST-vector magnitude (ST-VM) at 20 milliseconds after the termination of the QRS complex. These authors demonstrated a modest correlation between the ultimate QRS-VD and the maximal cumulative CK
release ($r = 0.64$) (Figure 2) and showed that the maximal spatial ST-
VM correlated with the ultimate QRS-VD ($r = 0.80$) (Figure 3). The
authors postulated the use of ultimate QRS-VD and maximal spatial ST-
VM as measures of ultimate infarct size. This opinion was supported
further by the good correlation between the cumulative myoglobin release after infarction and both the ultimate QRS-VD ($r = 0.85$) and the

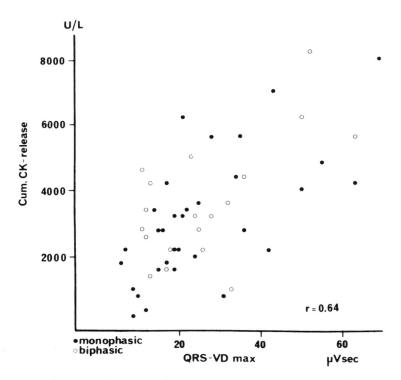

Figure 2. Relationship between ultimate creatine kinase (CK_{max}) and QRS vector
difference maximum ($QRS\text{-}VD_{max}$). The regression equation for all patients is

$$CK_{max} = 75.5 \times QRS\text{-}VD_{max} + 1330.$$

(Reproduced with permission from Reference 3.)

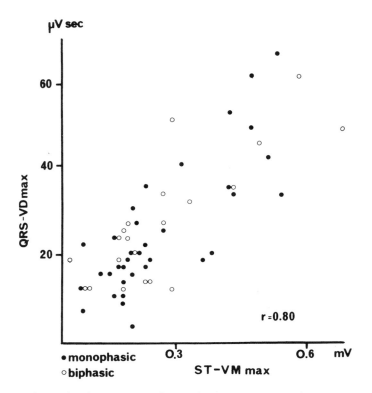

Figure 3. Relationship between initial spatial ST vector magnitude (ST-VM) and final maximal QRS vector differences (QRS-VD) in 56 patients. The regression equation is

$$\text{QRS-VD}_{max} = 72.8 \times \text{ST-VD}_{max} + 7.0.$$

(Reproduced with permission from Reference 3.)

initial spatial ST-VM ($r = 0.78$) (Figure 4).[4] Using this technique, Sederholm and coworkers[5] also showed that a cumulative pain score correlated positively with ultimate QRS-VD (Figure 5).

Dellborg et al[6] developed a continuous vectorcardiographic system (MIDA, Myocardial Infarction Diagnosis and Analysis, Ortivus Medical AB, Täby, Sweden) for automatically quantifying and displaying the QRS-VD and the ST-VM. These authors also described the variable patterns in the evolution of the QRS-VD and the ST-VM (Figure 6). Modest correlations were evident between total CK release and ultimate QRS-VD ($r = 0.44$) and ST-VM at 20 milliseconds ($r = 0.5$). ST-VM at 20 milliseconds correlated with ultimate QRS-VD ($r = 0.52$).

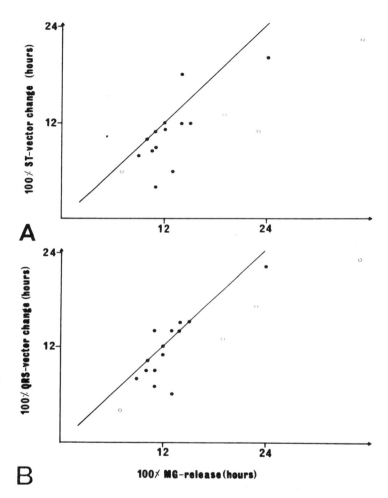

Figure 4. A. Correlation between the intervals (hours) between onset of symptoms and peak ST-vector change and onset of symptoms and peak myoglobin (MG) release. **B.** Correlation between time of peak QRS-vector change and peak MG release. **Solid circles** = survivors; **clear circles** = nonsurvivors. (Reproduced with permission from Reference 4.)

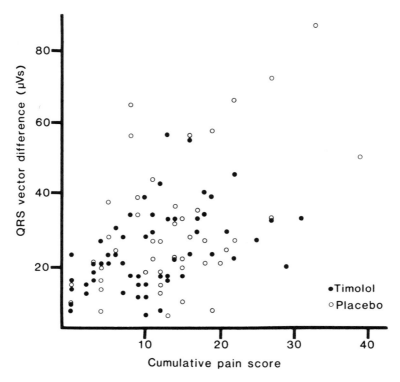

Figure 5. Correlation ($r = 0.51$) between cumulative chest pain score and maximal QRS-vector difference. (Reproduced with permission from Reference 5.)

Further support for the ability of vectorcardiographic data to quantify myocardial necrosis was provided by Dellborg et al,[7] who found that the ultimate QRS-VD at 24 hours correlated with enzymatic estimates of infarct size by lactate dehydrogenase-I, with r values between 0.52 and 0.68 depending on the site of infarction. This relationship between lactate dehydrogenase-I and ultimate QRS-VD was also present in patients receiving thrombolysis.[8] This latter study also showed a moderate correlation between ultimate QRS-VD and the ejection fraction 30 days after infarction ($r = 0.49$).

In addition, Dellborg et al[8] demonstrated a moderate correlation between initial ST-VM and lactate dehydrogenase-I ($r = 0.63$). Lundin et al[9] also showed an excellent correlation between the ultimate QRS-VD and maximal CK release ($r = 0.89$).

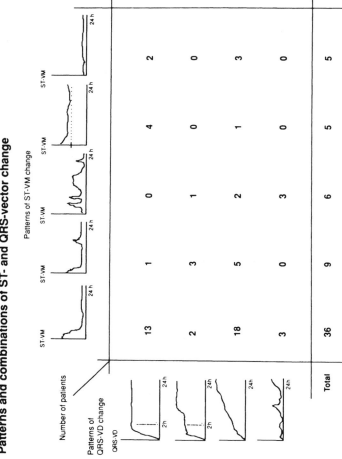

Figure 6. Patterns of QRS vector difference (QRS-VD) and ST-vector magnitude (ST-VM). The number of patients in each category is given. (Reproduced with permission from Reference 6.)

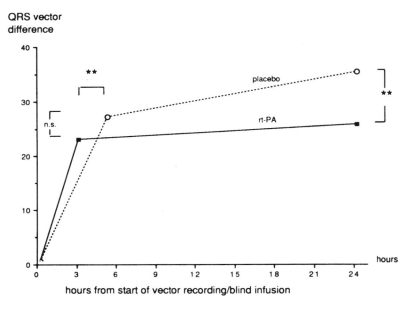

Figure 7. Rate of development of QRS-vector difference in patients receiving placebo and those receiving tissue plasminogen activator (rt-PA). NS = not significant; ** = $P<0.01$. (Reproduced with permission from Reference 8.)

Determination of Patency

Another use for continuous vectorcardiographic recording is the determination of coronary artery patency following thrombolysis. Dellborg et al[8] described the development of the QRS-VD with time in patients receiving tissue plasminogen activator. These authors noted that the ultimate QRS-VD occurred 131 minutes earlier in patients who had received thrombolysis than in those who had received placebo (Figure 7). Lundin et al[9] also noted the earlier development of the ultimate QRS-VD in patients who received streptokinase than in those who did not.

Strandberg et al[10] studied the QRS-VD in patients with acute evolving infarction treated with streptokinase. These authors also noted that stabilization of the QRS-VD occurred 4 hours earlier in the group that received streptokinase than in the group that did not. In addition, the ST-VM declined to a plateau some 2 hours earlier in the treated group (Figure 8). This pattern was also reflected in the earlier termination of myoglobin and CK-MB release in the patients who received streptokinase.

Dellborg et al[11] demonstrated that rapid evolution of the vectorcardiographic variables, QRS-VD and ST-VM, was associated with a high angiographic patency of the infarct-related artery following thrombolysis (Figure 9A). The converse was true if the infarct-related artery remained occluded after thrombolysis (Figure 9B). Furthermore, Dellborg et al,[12] using the QRS-VD and ST-VM, were able to distinguish between streptokinase and tissue plasminogen activator. The QRS-VD reached a plateau earlier in patients who received tissue plasminogen activator than in those who received streptokinase. However, the ST-VM recovery and the size of the ultimate QRS-VD were not different between the tissue plasminogen activator (alteplase) group and the streptokinase group (Figure 10). These authors interpreted the data to mean that patency occurred earlier with tissue plasminogen activator, but that final infarct size did not differ between the treatment groups. However, angiographic confirmation of infarct-related artery patency was not available in these patients. The more rapid development of both the ultimate QRS-VD and the minimal ST-VM could also represent completion of necrosis rather than myocardial salvage with reperfusion.

Early Vectorcardiographic Features

Another vectorcardiographic feature used to quantify myocardial infarction was found in the initial portion of the QRS signal. Cowan et al[13,14] noted that the first derivative of the QRS complex in the X, Y, and Z leads had an unusual feature related to myocardial infarct size. This feature was termed the "initial period of abnormal depolarization" (IAD). The IAD, when analyzed on the first derivative graph, terminated with a distinct downslope or notch (Figure 11A). In normal subjects, an early period of slower depolarization is seen (Figure 11B). This was thought to correspond to the IAD seen in patients with myocardial infarction. The sum of the integrals of the IAD in the vectorcardiographic leads was much greater in patients with infarction than in normal subjects. These authors showed that this abnormality could be used to detect infarction and to quantify myocardial infarction in postmortem studies (Figure 12).[13–15] These analyses also showed that late activation information in the QRS could be obtained in a similar manner and did contribute to the measurement of infarct size, particularly in inferobasal infarction.[15] Cowan and colleagues[16] have shown that the initial area of depolarization was less in patients who received streptokinase than in a control group.

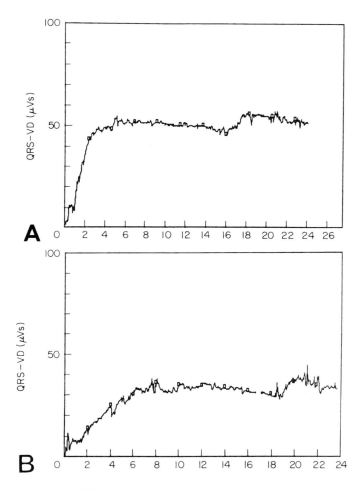

Figure 8. QRS-vector difference (QRS-VD, **A** and **B**) and ST-vector magnitude at 20 milliseconds (ST-VM20, **C** and **D**) in patients with acute myocardial infarction treated with streptokinase with reperfusion (**A** and **C**) and without reperfusion (**B** and **D**). (Reproduced with permission from Reference 10.)

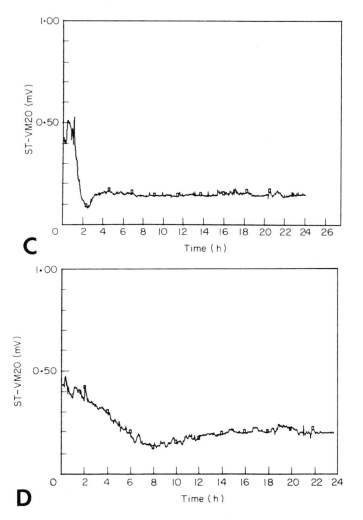

Figure 8. *(continued)*

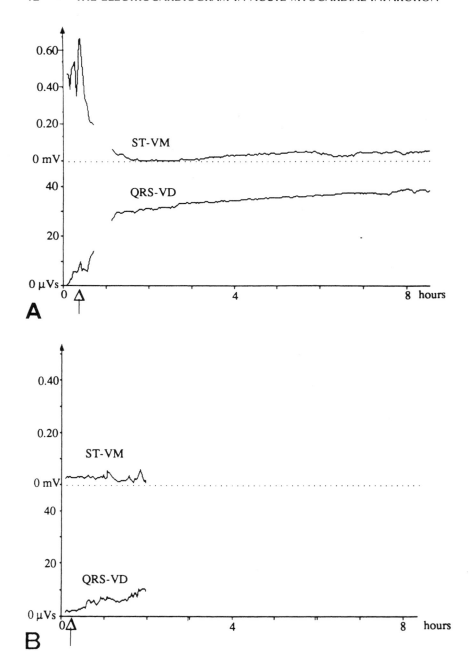

Other Vectorcardiographic Features and Myocardial Infarction

The vectorcardiographic loops have been explored as an estimate of infarct size. Morikawa et al[17] examined indentations, or "bites," in the vector loops occurring in dogs after experimental myocardial infarction (Figure 13). The duration of the bite correlated with the size of the infarct ($r = 0.67$) (Figure 14A). The QRS-VD measured in the same study also correlated with infarct size ($r = 0.71$) (Figure 14B).

Change in the vector loop after infarction was used by Selvester and Sanmarco[18] to quantify myocardial infarction in humans. These investigators used vector loops in the three orthogonal planes both before and after infarction in a group of 74 patients. The change in the loops after infarction was measured by two variables. The first was the duration of the abnormality and the second was the maximal magnitude in millivolts of the change in vector. The values analyzed were those with the greatest value in any of the three orthogonal planes. These authors were able to generate a nomogram that related these vectorcardiographic variables to angiographic determinants of infarct size, such as left ventricular ejection fraction and extent of wall motion abnormality (Figure 15).

Vectorcardiography and Prognosis After Infarction

Recently, continuous on-line vectorcardiographic recordings in the intensive care unit have been used to study prognosis after myocardial infarction. Lundin et al[19] studied 203 patients with acute myocardial infarction in whom continuous vectorcardiographic recordings were initiated immediately upon arrival in the intensive care unit and maintained for 24 hours. These patients were followed for a mean ($\pm$ SD) of 538 ($\pm$ 220) days. Of these 203 patients, 36 (18%) died (6 during hospitalization) and 38 (19%) were hospitalized for reinfarction (13 were fatal reinfarctions). These authors demonstrated two patterns of QRS-VD and ST-VM in these patients. The first pattern (Figure 16A) showed multiple transient changes in the QRS-VD and ST-VM, and the second pattern showed rapid development of the QRS-VD to a plateau and rapid decrease in the ST-VM to baseline (Figure 16B)., Nonsurvi-

◄──────────────────────────────────────

Figure 9. ST-vector magnitude (ST-VM) and QRS-vector difference (QRS-VD) in two patients with acute myocardial infarction with either pharmacologic reperfusion (**A**) or persistent infarct-related artery occlusion (**B**). **Arrow** = angiography. (Reproduced with permission from Reference 11.)

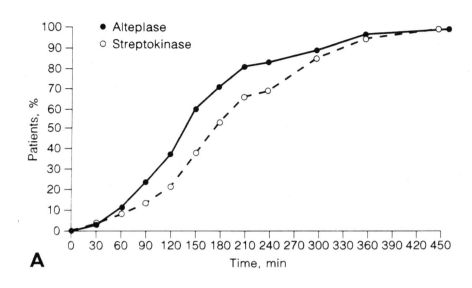

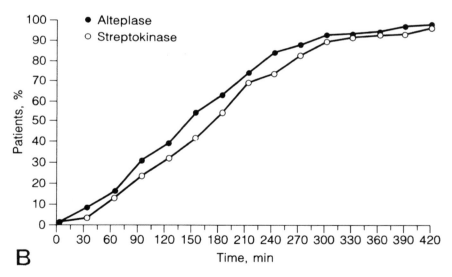

Figure 10. Cumulative percentages of patients with acute infarction who have reached a plateau in the QRS-vector difference (**A**) or the ST-vector magnitude (**B**) with acute infarction treated with either tissue plasminogen activator (alteplase) (•) or streptokinase (o). (Reproduced with permission from Reference 12.)

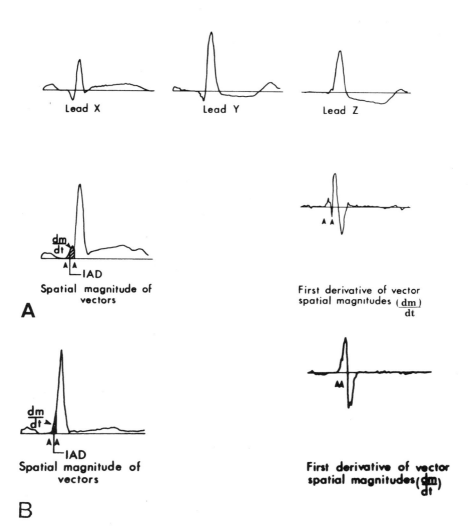

Figure 11. A. Computer printout of leads X, Y, and Z in patients with acute myocardial infarction. The spatial magnitude of the vectors and the rate of change with time of the spatial magnitude are shown. The initial abnormal depolarization (IAD) is shown by the **cross-hatched area. B.** The spatial magnitude of the vectors and the rate of change with time of the spatial magnitude in a normal subject. (Reproduced with permission from Reference 14.)

MI's and Controls

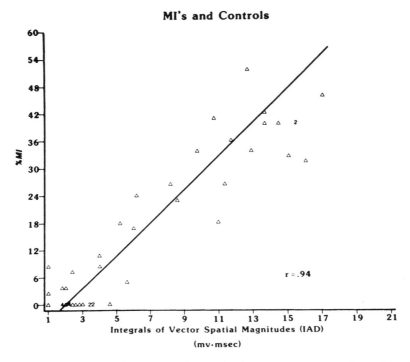

Figure 12. Correlation of percent volume of infarction (%MI) as estimated by left ventriculography (y-axis) and integral of spatial vector magnitude during the initial abnormal depolarization (IAD, x-axis). %MI = $-4.55 + 3.62$ IAD; $r = 0.94$. (Reproduced with permission from Reference 15.)

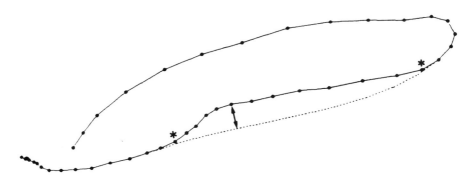

Figure 13. A QRS loop with a "bite" (in a dog with a ligated coronary artery). * indicates the start and end of the bite. **Arrow** indicates the amplitude of the bite. (Reproduced with permission from Reference 17.)

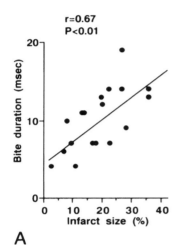

A

Figure 14. **A.** Scatterplot of bite duration and infarct size. **B.** Scatterplot of QRS-vector difference (QRS-VD) and infarct size. The data were obtained in dogs 6 hours after ligation of the coronary artery. (Reproduced with permission from Reference 17.)

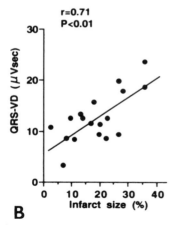

B

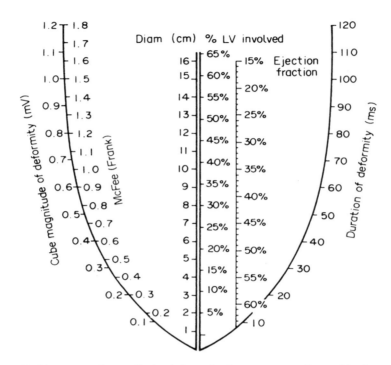

Figure 15. Nomogram for predicting infarct size from vectorcardiographic abnormalities. (Reproduced with permission from Startt/Selvester RH, Wagner GS, Ideker RE: Myocardial infarction. In: Macfarlane PW, Veitch Lawrie TD (eds): *Comprehensive Electrocardiology: Theory and Practice in Health and Disease.* Vol 1. New York: Pergamon Press; 565–629, 1989 as adapted from Reference 18.)

vors were more likely to have multiple episodes of transient changes in QRS-VD and ST-VM than survivors. Also, survivors were more likely to have rapid development of the QRS-VD and decrease in the ST-VM (Figure 17).

Lundin et al[19] thought that multiple transient changes in the QRS-VD and ST-VM represented multiple episodes of transient myocardial ischemia, whereas the rapid development of the QRS-VD and increase

Figure 16. A. Trend curves in QRS-vector difference (QRS-VD) and change in ST-vector magnitude (STC-VM) in a patient with subendocardial infarction. The transient changes in the QRS and ST variables are thought to be due to ischemic episodes during evolution of acute infarction. **B.** Pattern of rapid increase in QRS-VD and rapid decrease in ST-VM seen in a patient receiving streptokinase. This pattern is suggested to show reperfusion. (Reproduced with permission from Reference 19.)

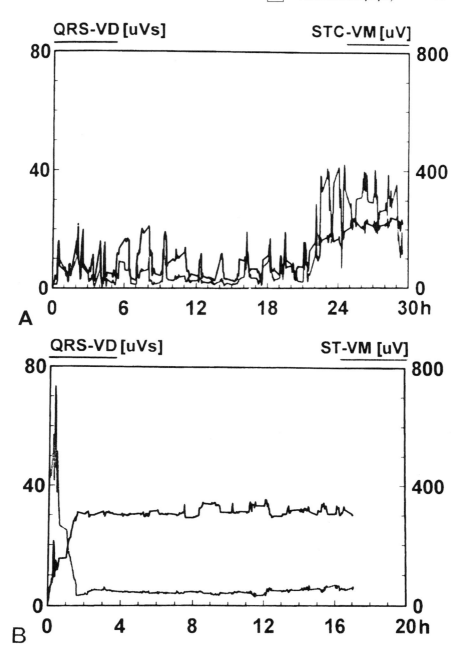

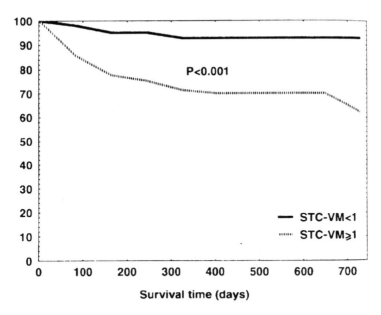

Figure 17. Cumulative survival (Kaplan-Meier method) for patients with and for those without transient changes of ST change-vector magnitude (STC-VM). (Reproduced with permission from Reference 19.)

in the ST-VM were associated with reperfusion. They provided criteria for myocardial ischemia as a reversible increase in QRS-VD by >15 microvolt seconds from the previous measure of QRS-VD lasting for 2 minutes or more, and a reversible increase in ST-VM by >0.05 mV from the preceding ST-VM lasting for 2 minutes or more. When both of these variables were present, failed reperfusion was said to be present. In multivariate analysis, this criterion for failed reperfusion, the ultimate QRS-VD, and episodes of ST-VM, predicted mortality with a r^2 of 42.8, and these variables had independent predictive prognostic ability compared with age, sex, maximal CK value, chest radiographic findings, heart size, occurrence of ventricular fibrillation, and inability to perform exercise testing. The combination of the vectorcardiographic data and clinical data yielded a model with increased predictive value ($r^2 = 81.1$). These authors thought that continuous monitoring with vectorcardiography could be used to identify patients at high risk and, thus, to select patients for early angiography or intervention (or both).

Summary

Multiple variables obtained from vectorcardiographic recordings can be used to quantify the size of a myocardial infarct. Features from the

X, Y, and Z leads include QRS-VD, the initial period of depolarization, and the late period of depolarization. The ST-VM in the early hours after infarction can be used to predict final infarct size. The vector loops also give information. Indentations in the loops or the magnitude and extent of the loop distortions after infarction are correlated with infarct size.

With regard to prediction of reperfusion, continuous vectorcardiographic recording is valuable. In particular, early stabilization of the QRS-VD and ST-VM changes are predictors of reperfusion. In addition, multiple changes in the QRS-VD and ST-VM indicate an adverse prognosis and, if detected within 24 hours after hospital admission, may indicate a subgroup of patients that requires early angiography and consideration of revascularization.

Thus, vectorcardiography has considerable potential for studying acute myocardial infarction and interventions designed to limit infarction. However, more studies are needed in which all these variables are measured in the setting of reperfusion and infarct quantification. This approach truly will evaluate the role of vectorcardiography in the management of acute infarction.

References

1. Hodges M, Akiyama T, Biddle TL, Clarke WB, Roberts DL, Kronenberg MW: Continuous recording of the vectorcardiogram in acutely ill patients. *Am Heart J* 88:593–595, 1974.
2. Wikswo JP Jr, Gundersen SC, Murphy W, Dawson AK, Smith RF: Sequential QRS vector subtractions in acute myocardial infarction in humans. Time course and relationship to serial changes in serum CK-MB concentration. *Circ Res* 49: 1055–1062, 1981.
3. Sederholm M, Grottum P, Erhardt L, Kjekshus J: Quantitative assessment of myocardial ischemia and necrosis by continuous vectorcardiography and measurement of creatine kinase release in patients. *Circulation* 68:1006–1012, 1983.
4. Sederholm M, Sylven C: Relation between ST and QRS vector changes and myoglobin release in acute myocardial infarction. *Cardiovasc Res* 17:589–594, 1983.
5. Sederholm M, Grottum P, Kjekshus J, Erhardt L: Course of chest pain and its relation to CK release and ST/QRS vector changes in patients with acute myocardial infarction randomized to treatment with intravenous timolol or placebo. *Am Heart J* 110:521–528, 1985.
6. Dellborg M, Riha M, Swedberg K: Dynamic QRS and ST-segment changes in myocardial infarction monitored by continuous on-line vectorcardiography. *J Electrocardiol* 23(suppl):11–19, 1990.
7. Dellborg M, Herlitz J, Risenfors M, Swedberg K: Electrocardiographic assessment of infarct size: comparison between QRS scoring of 12-lead electrocardiography and dynamic vectorcardiography. *Int J Cardiol* 40:167–172, 1993.
8. Dellborg M, Riha M, Swedberg K: Dynamic QRS-complex and ST-segment monitoring in acute myocardial infarction during recombinant tissue-type plasminogen activator therapy. *Am J Cardiol* 67:343–349, 1991.

9. Lundin P, Eriksson SV, Erhardt L, Strandberg LE, Rehnqvist N: Continuous vectorcardiography in patients with chest pain indicative of acute ischemic heart disease. *Cardiology* 81:145–156, 1992.
10. Strandberg LE, Sylven C, Erhardt L: Continuous ST- and QRS-vector changes and myoglobin release during streptokinase-treated acute myocardial infarction. *Eur Heart J* 13:511–516, 1992.
11. Dellborg M, Topol EJ, Swedberg K: Dynamic QRS complex and ST-segment vectorcardiographic monitoring can identify vessel patency in patients with acute myocardial infarction treated with reperfusion therapy. *Am Heart J* 122:943–948, 1991.
12. Dellborg M, Svensson AM, Johansson M, Swedberg K: Early electrocardiographic changes in acute myocardial infarction treated by streptokinase or alteplase: a randomized study with dynamic, multilead, electrocardiographic monitoring. *Cardiology* 82:368–376, 1993.
13. Cowan MJ, Reichenbach DD, Bruce RA, Fisher L: Estimation of myocardial infarct size by digital computer analysis of the VCG. *J Electrocardiol* 15:307–316, 1982.
14. Cowan MJ, Bruce RA, Van Winkle D, Davidson L, Killpack A: Comparative accuracy of computerized spatial vectorcardiography and standard electrocardiography for detection of myocardial infarction. *J Electrocardiol* 18:111–122, 1985.
15. Cowan MJ, Bruce RA, Reichenbach DD: Validation of a computerized QRS criterion for estimating myocardial infarction size and correlation with quantitative morphologic measurements. *Am J Cardiol* 57:60–65, 1986.
16. Cowan M, Hindman N, Wagner G, Ritchie J, Cerqueira M: Estimation of myocardial infarct size by electrocardiographic and radionuclide techniques. *J Electrocardiol* 20(suppl):78–81, 1987.
17. Morikawa J, Furukawa T, Tanaka H, et al: Analysis of bites on three-dimensional vectorcardiography after coronary artery ligation in dogs. *J Electrocardiol* 24:387–394, 1991.
18. Selvester RH, Sanmarco M: Infarct size in hi-gain hi-fidelity serial VCG's and serial ventriculograms in patients with proven coronary artery disease. Excerpta Medica International Congress Series No. 444: 523–528, 1977.
19. Lundin P, Eriksson SV, Strandberg LE, Rehnqvist N: Prognostic information from on-line vectorcardiography in acute myocardial infarction. *Am J Cardiol* 74:1103–1108, 1994.

Precordial Electrocardiographic Mapping

Ian P. Clements, MD

Introduction

Precordial electrocardiographic (ECG) mapping as a measure of the extent of myocardium that is at risk of infarction or the extent of myocardial infarction is derived from experimental studies that used epicardial ECGs as a way of measuring these variables.

Several aspects of the epicardial ECG have been studied. Hillis et al[1] assessed the relationship of changes in R-wave height and Q-wave depth at specific epicardial sites to myocardial cell damage at these sites 24 hours after ligation of the coronary artery. They showed that the sum of the change in R-wave height and Q-wave depth of the epicardial ECG was negatively correlated with loss of myocardial creatine kinase (CK-MB) (Figure 1) and histologic grade of necrosis seen at these sites ($r = -0.86 \pm 0.03$). To obtain an estimate of the change in R wave and Q wave 24 hours after coronary artery occlusion, the authors assessed the ST-segment elevation at the corresponding sites 15 minutes after arterial occlusion and found a reasonable correlation ($r = 0.8 \pm 0.06$) between these variables. Hillis et al[1] believed that the ST-segment elevation at a particular epicardial site 15 minutes after coronary occlusion was a reasonable predictor of the final degree of myocardial damage at that site. In this study, the authors demonstrated that the administration of hyaluronidase or propranolol 20 minutes after coronary artery occlusion caused a significant reduction in the Q wave and R wave at 24 hours in comparison with the anticipated Q wave and R wave based on the ST-segment elevation at 15 minutes (Figure 2).

From: Clements, IP (ed). *The Electrocardiogram in Acute Myocardial Infarction.* Armonk, NY: Futura Publishing Company, Inc. © Mayo Foundation 1998.

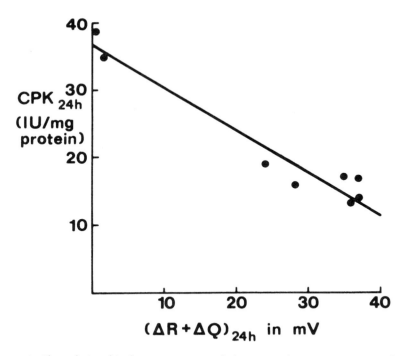

Figure 1. The relationship between myocardial creatine kinase (CPK) at 24 hours after experimental infarction in a dog and the change in the sum of R and Q waves ($\Delta R + \Delta Q$) at the site of myocardial CPK sampling. The correlation between CPK and $\Delta R + \Delta Q$ is negative. (Reproduced with permission from Reference 1.)

An important experimental study was performed by Muller and colleagues.[2] One of their goals was to determine whether the precordial ECG could substitute for the epicardial ECG. This study, performed in dogs, reported on simultaneous QRS and ST mapping from both an epicardial and a precordial array of 30 electrodes after occlusion of the left anterior descending coronary artery. The authors identified a close correlation ($r = 0.92 \pm 0.01$) between summated epicardial and precordial ST-segment elevation after coronary artery occlusion. This correlation was present during intermittent coronary artery occlusion and after administering isoproterenol and propranolol. The summated value of both epicardial and precordial ST-segment elevation 15 to 30 minutes after occlusion was related to tissue levels of CK 24 hours later; marked ST-segment elevation was associated with considerable CK loss and myocardial necrosis, and little ST-segment elevation was associated with myocardial preservation. Also, normalization of precordial and epicardial ST-segment elevation after reperfusion was associated with myocardial preservation. Changes in both epicardial and precordial R-wave height 15 to 60 minutes after occlusion or reperfusion were also related to myocardial necrosis and viability 24 hours later.

Muller et al[2] emphasized an important source for error in this technique, namely, the occurrence of conduction delay in the center of large areas of ischemia (Figure 3). This conduction delay causes a widening in the QRS complex and a decrease in ST-segment elevation. The decrease in ST-segment elevation in these circumstances is associated paradoxically with profound ischemia. These authors recommended that

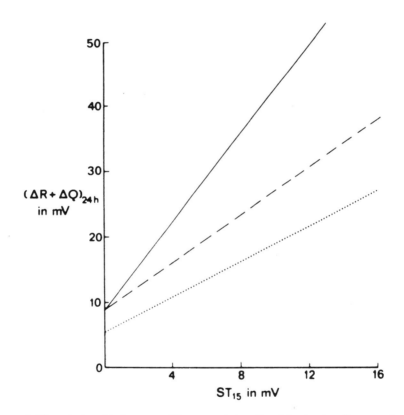

Figure 2. The relationship between ST-segment elevation 15 minutes after experimental occlusion and changes in QRS configuration 24 hours after occlusion [(ΔR + ΔQ)$_{24 h}$]. **Solid line** represents the control group of dogs. **Dotted line** indicates the group of dogs that received hyaluronidase. **Dashed line** represents the group of dogs that received propranolol. Note that for the propranolol and hyaluronidase groups of dogs, a given ST-segment elevation at 15 minutes was associated with a lesser degree of change in QRS configuration, reflecting less myocardial necrosis. (Reproduced with permission from Reference 1.)

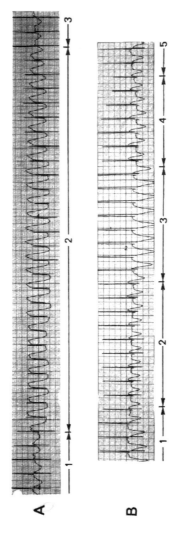

Figure 3. Epicardial ECGs obtained with an electrode swept across an area of myocardial infarction in two dogs. **A.** ST-segment elevation progresses to a peak value from the edge of the infarct to the middle. **B.** ST-segment elevation declines from the edge to the center of the infarct and the QRS widens. This indicates the phenomenon of infarction block. When QRS widening occurs in the setting of acute infarction, ST-segment measurements cannot be used to estimate the degree of myocardial ischemia. (Reproduced with permission from Reference 2.)

ECGs that show QRS prolongation be excluded from this type of quantitative analysis.

Application of Precordial Mapping to Humans

Askenazi et al[3] summated the R-wave height from standard 12-lead ECGs and demonstrated a decrease in R-wave height with time after acute myocardial infarction.

Precordial ECG maps have been used in several ways to quantify myocardial infarction in humans. For example, an ECG variable, such as R-wave height or ST-segment height, can be summated over all the leads of the precordial array. These variables can then be correlated with infarct size or arterial patency.

Another method of using the array is to define the precordial area over which a certain ECG finding is present. This could be the precordial area of the presence of pathologic Q waves or the precordial area of

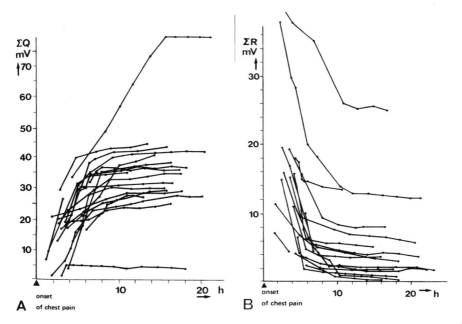

Figure 4. A. Spontaneous course of Q-wave development in 20 patients admitted to a coronary care unit early after the onset of chest pain. **B.** Spontaneous decline of R waves during the first hours of the onset of myocardial infarction. (Reproduced with permission from Reference 4.)

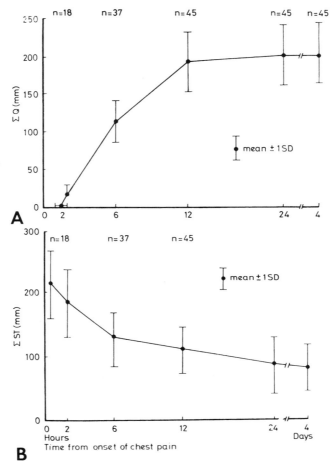

Figure 5. A. The sum of the Q waves (ΣQ) at intervals, up to 4 days, after the onset of symptoms of infarction in patients with anterior infarction. **B.** The sum of ST-segment elevation (ΣST) at intervals, up to 4 days, after the onset of symptoms of infarction in patients with anterior infarction. (Reproduced with permission from Reference 5.)

a certain degree of ST-segment elevation. The precordial area is then correlated with infarct size or arterial patency.

Precordial mapping has been performed in patients with evolving myocardial infarction. In 1980, von Essen et al[4] used a precordial array of 48 electrodes to describe the serial changes in summated Q wave and R wave in 42 patients with evolving anterior myocardial infarction. The

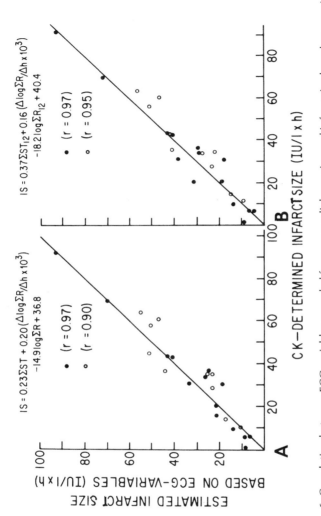

Figure 6. Correlation between ECG variables recorded from precordial mapping and infarct size based on creatine kinase (CK)-determined infarct size. The ECG variables are ΣST, log ΣR, and ($\Delta log\ \Sigma R/\Delta hour$) 10^3. **A.** Graph is from the initial recorded values. **B.** Graph is from time-corrected values. **Solid circles** indicate initial study group of 14 patients; **open circles** represent validation group of 10 patients. (Reproduced with permission from Reference 6.)

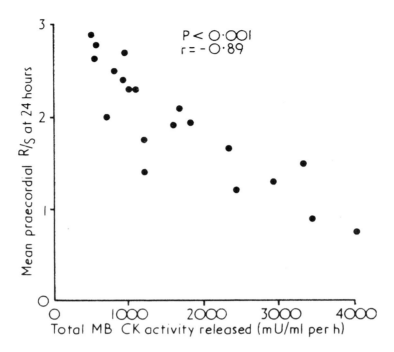

Figure 7. Relationship between the R/S ratio observed on a precordial map and the total creatine kinase (CK) released. (Reproduced with permission from Reference 7.)

Q- and R-wave magnitudes increased and declined, respectively, over about a 10-hour period after the onset of the symptoms of infarction and reached a plateau that remained constant unless reinfarction occurred (Figure 4). If there was reinfarction, further loss of the R wave or increase in the Q wave occurred. On the basis of these data, von Essen et al[4] believed that interventions to alter the course of infarction must occur before the ECG changes are complete. Selwyn et al[5] recorded precordial maps (72 electrodes) of Q waves and ST-segment elevation in 45 patients with evolving myocardial infarction and showed that Q waves often developed within 2 hours after the onset of symptoms and that changes in the precordial measures had developed fully by 12 hours, well before peak plasma activity of CK-MB was reached (Figure 5).

Application of Precordial Mapping to Estimation of Infarct Size and Area at Risk in Humans

Henning et al[6] studied changes in summated ST-segment elevation and R wave from 35 precordial leads in 24 patients with uncomplicated anterior myocardial infarction. QRS complexes were not allowed to exceed 90 milliseconds in duration. They derived a model that included the summated ST segment, the summated R wave, and the decline in R-wave height and that was able to predict quite accurately final infarct size ($r = 0.97$) as estimated from serial serum measurements of levels of CK (Figure 6). The authors were hopeful that this approach would be applicable to the study of the effects of interventions.

Selwyn et al[7] studied the mean ratio of R and S waves recorded from a 72-electrode precordial array in 45 patients with acute anterior myocardial infarction. This study showed a good correlation ($r = 0.89$) between the mean R/S ratio at 24 hours after the onset of symptoms and total MB CK released (Figure 7).

Selwyn et al[5] also analyzed the precordial ECG signal in terms of the precordial area with a specific abnormality. They demonstrated that the precordial area of ST-segment elevation at 45 and 120 minutes correlated ($r = 0.95$ and 0.88, respectively) with the precordial area of Q-wave development at 24 hours (Figure 8).

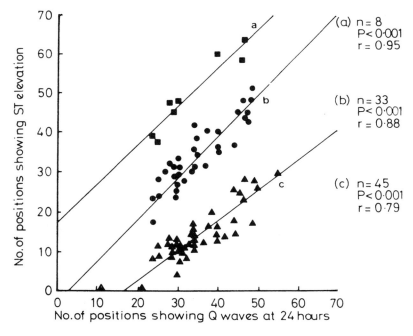

Figure 8. Relationships between ST-segment elevation (y-axis) at (**a**) 45 minutes, (**b**) 2 hours, and (**c**) 12 hours and Q-wave area at 24 hours. The ST-segment elevation at these various times can be used to predict final infarct size as estimated from the Q wave. (Reproduced with permission from Reference 5.)

Selwyn et al[8] extended their studies of precordial mapping by assessing the effect of early administration of methylprednisolone; this study also included a control group of patients with anterior infarction. The authors demonstrated an excellent correlation (r, between 0.91 and 0.92) of the relationship between the extent of precordial ST-segment elevation at 2 to 3 hours, 5 to 6 hours, and 12 hours after the onset of symptoms, and the extent of precordial Q-wave development at 24 hours. The administration of methylprednisolone was associated with an attenuation of the development of precordial Q waves at 24 hours as predicted by the precordial ST-segment distribution early after the onset of symptoms (Figure 9).

Yusuf et al,[9] using a 35-lead system, analyzed the ability of early precordial mapping to predict and to measure final infarct size; both summated ECG variables and the precordial area of ECG abnormality

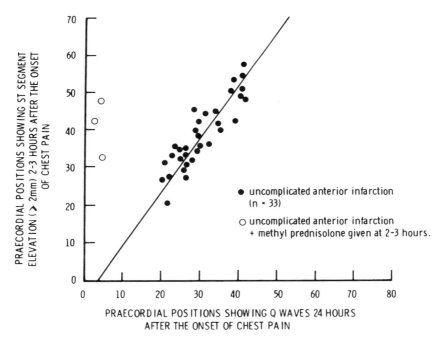

Figure 9. Influence of methylprednisolone on the relationship between ST-segment elevation at 2 to 3 hours and Q waves at 24 hours. Early administration of methylprednisolone led to considerable decrease in the final Q-wave extent compared with the initial ST-segment elevation. Thus, methylprednisolone decreased final infarct size as compared with the area at risk for infarction. (Reproduced with permission from Reference 8.)

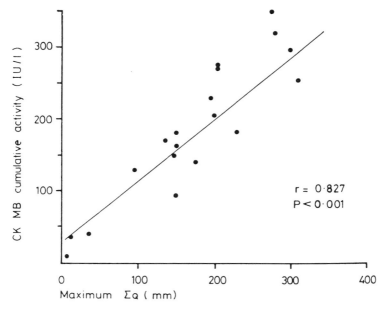

Figure 10. Maximum ΣQ from precordial mapping (x-axis) and cumulative creatine kinase (CK-MB) activity (y-axis) in patients with anterior infarction. The correlation of 0.827 is highly significant ($P<0.001$). (Reproduced with permission from Reference 9.)

were assessed. The authors found that there was an excellent correlation ($r = 0.827$) between the maximal summated precordial Q wave observed over a 3-day period and the final infarct size as estimated by cumulative CK-MB release (Figure 10). The maximal summated ST-segment elevation was reasonably correlated ($r = 0.733$) with cumulative CK-MB release. Yusuf et al[9] also found a good correlation ($r = 0.820$) between maximal summated ST-segment elevation and maximal summated Q-wave depth. One of the points the authors emphasized was that these results were true only for anterior infarction. Also, they believed that the summated ST-segment elevation and Q-wave magnitudes, rather than the number of leads showing ST-segment elevation or Q-waves, correlated better with the final infarct size as determined by cumulative CK-MB. The authors showed that in inferior infarction, the sum of the maximal Q waves in leads II, III, and aVF correlated ($r = 0.745$) with cumulative CK-MB release (Figure 11); the correlation with summated ST-segment elevation in these leads was less striking ($r = 0.505$), and the summated ST-segment elevation and Q-wave depth did not correlate.

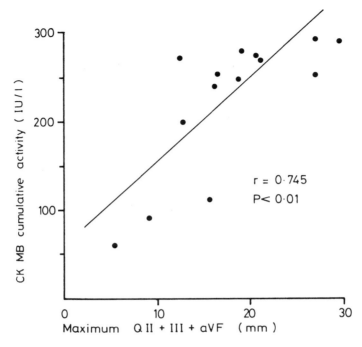

Figure 11. ΣQ in leads II, III, and aVF plotted against cumulative creatine kinase (CK-MB) release in patients with inferior infarction. (Reproduced with permission from Reference 9.)

Assessment of Reperfusion With Precordial Mapping

Attempts have been made to use precordial mapping to identify reperfusion. Kilpatrick et al[10] suggested that within 2 hours after the onset of the symptoms of infarction, reversal of the ST pattern on precordial maps after thrombolysis suggest reperfusion. However, only 15 of the 66 patients in the study were assessed during this time interval. Also, conclusions about the value of precordial mapping in detecting reperfusion in acute myocardial infarction cannot be drawn from this study because early angiography was not performed.

Limitations of Precordial Mapping

Major limitations of precordial mapping are related to the cumbersome nature of the equipment. It is necessary to record ECGs from multiple leads simultaneously. This becomes more difficult when serial recordings are necessary. Certainly, this is somewhat easier when fixed arrays of electrodes are used rather than multiple electrodes.

Another difficulty is related to the recording and analysis of the data, the identification of specific points to analyze, and the presentation of the data. Certainly, computer storage and display of the data make recording, analyzing, and presenting the data easier. Additional problems are related to the genesis of the ECG, in particular the determinants of ST-segment changes. The changes in ST and R wave induced by the development of intramyocardial block are mentioned above.[2] However, the ST segment is sensitive to many changes, such as pericarditis, alteration in electrolyte concentration, variation in heart rate, and medications. Also, the precordial mapping method for quantification of infarction may be limited to patients with anterior infarction.

References

1. Hillis LD, Askenazi J, Braunwald E, et al: Use of changes in the epicardial QRS complex to assess interventions which modify the extent of myocardial necrosis following coronary artery occlusion. *Circulation* 54:591–598, 1976.
2. Muller JE, Maroko PR, Braunwald E: Evaluation of precordial electrocardiographic mapping as a means of assessing changes in myocardial ischemic injury. *Circulation* 52:16–27, 1975.
3. Askenazi J, Maroko PR, Lesch M, Braunwald E: Usefulness of ST segment elevations as predictors of electrocardiographic signs of necrosis in patients with acute myocardial infarction. *Br Heart J* 39:764–770, 1977.
4. von Essen R, Merx W, Doerr R, Effert S, Silny J, Rau G: QRS mapping in the evaluation of acute anterior myocardial infarction. *Circulation* 62:266–276, 1980.
5. Selwyn AP, Fox K, Welman E, Shillingford JP: Natural history and evaluation of Q waves during acute myocardial infarction. *Br Heart J* 40:383–387, 1978.
6. Henning H, Hardarson T, Francis G, O'Rourke RA, Ryan W, Ross J Jr: Approach to the estimation of myocardial infarct size by analysis of precordial S-T segment and R wave maps. *Am J Cardiol* 41:1–8, 1978.
7. Selwyn AP, Ogunro E, Shillingford JP: Loss of electrically active myocardium during anterior infarction in man. *Br Heart J* 39:1186–1191, 1977.
8. Selwyn AP, Fox KM, Welman E, Jonathan A, Shillingford JP: Electrocardiographic precordial mapping in anterior myocardial infarction. The critical period for interventions as exemplified by methylprednisolone. *Circulation* 58:892–897, 1978.
9. Yusuf S, Lopez R, Maddison A, et al: Value of electrocardiogram in predicting and estimating infarct size in man. *Br Heart J* 42:286–293, 1979.
10. Kilpatrick D, Bell AJ, Briggs C: Assessment of reperfusion in myocardial infarction by body surface electrocardiographic mapping. *J Electrocardiol* 26:279–289, 1993.

4

Electrocardiographic Parameter Variability in Acute Myocardial Infarction

Stephen J. Pieper, MD

Optimal treatment of myocardial infarction requires establishing patency of the infarct-related artery and risk stratification, both in-hospital and after dismissal.[1] This chapter focuses on heart rate variability (HRV) as a tool to assess patency of the infarct-related artery, myocardial ischemia, and risk stratification early after myocardial infarction.

Heart Rate Variability

Beat-to-beat changes in HRV result in large part from the responsiveness of the sinoatrial node to alterations in autonomic tone.[2-8] Analysis of HRV has been reported most commonly in the "time domain" or "frequency domain."[9-14] Time-domain methods include calculation of signal averages, for example, mean heart rate, variance, and root mean square values.[11,14,15] Frequency-domain methods include calculation of frequency transforms such as low- and high-frequency spectral density.[5,12,15] Table 1 defines some frequently reported time- and frequency-domain analysis variables and gives their units of measure. The HRV power spectrum is obtained from the Fourier transform of an RR interval trend plot (Figure 1A). The power spectrum is represented graphically as variance (usually measured in ms^2/Hz or beats/minute) plotted against frequency (Figures 1B and 1C). Detailed descriptions

From: Clements, IP (ed). *The Electrocardiogram in Acute Myocardial Infarction.*
Armonk, NY: Futura Publishing Company, Inc. © Mayo Foundation 1998.

Table 1
Definition and Units of Measure of Some Heart Rate Variability Time and
Frequency Domain Variables

Variable	Domain	Units	Definition
Night-day difference	Time	ms	Difference between the average of all the normal RR intervals at night (24:00 to 05:00) and the average of all the normal RR intervals during the day (07:30 to 21:30)
SDNN	Time	ms	Standard deviation of all normal RR intervals in the entire 24-hour ECG recording
SDANN index	Time	ms	Standard deviation of the average normal RR intervals for all 5-minute segments of a 24-hour ECG recording (each average is weighted by the fraction of the 5 minutes that has normal RR intervals)
SDNN index	Time	ms	Mean of the standard deviations of all normal RR intervals for all 5-minute segments of a 24-hour ECG recording
r-MSSD	Time	ms	Root-mean-square successive difference (the square root of the mean of the squared differences between adjacent normal RR intervals over the entire 24-hour ECG recording)
pNN50	Time	%	Percentage of differences between adjacent normal RR intervals that are >50 ms computed over the entire 24-hour ECG recording
Total power	Frequency	ms^2	The energy in the heart period power spectrum up to 0.40 Hz
Ultralow-frequency power	Frequency	ms^2	The energy in the heart period power spectrum up to 0.0033 Hz
Very LF power	Frequency	ms^2	The energy in the heart period power spectrum between 0.0033 and 0.04 Hz
LF power	Frequency	ms^2	The energy in the heart period power spectrum between 0.04 and 0.15 Hz
HF power	Frequency	ms^2	The energy in the heart period power spectrum between 0.15 and 0.40 Hz
LF/HF ratio	Frequency	None	The ratio of low- to high-frequency power

ECG = electrocardiographic; HF = high frequency; LF = low frequency.

Reproduced with permission from Bigger JT Jr, Fleiss JL, Steinman RC, Rolnitzky LM, Kleiger RE, Rottman JN: Correlations among time and frequency domain measures of heart period variability two weeks after acute myocardial infarction. *Am J Cardiol* 69:891–898, 1992.

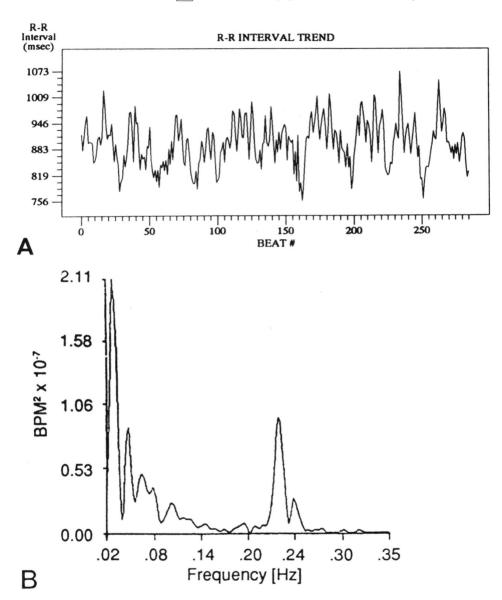

Figure 1. A. The beat-to-beat variability in RR cycle length expressed in milliseconds versus beat number. **B.** Spectral plot of variance in RR cycle length expressed in beats per minute squared (BPM^2) versus frequency from a "healthy" volunteer. This is often referred to as the "power spectrum."

of the techniques used to determine HRV signals from the surface electrocardiogram (ECG) have been reported extensively and are beyond the scope of this chapter. The interested reader is referred to several reports on this topic.[11–13,16–19]

Early analysis of HRV revealed three prominent peaks in the HRV power spectrum in a canine model: low-, mid-, and high-frequency peaks (Figure 2).[5] The size of the high-frequency peak (0.15–0.35 Hz) is thought to be directly proportional to the responsiveness of the sinoatrial node to alterations in its parasympathetic input.[5–8] The mid-, low-, very low-, and ultralow-frequency peaks are modulated largely by changes in sympathetic tone. However, parasympathetic tone and other physiologic and nonphysiologic inputs also affect this portion of

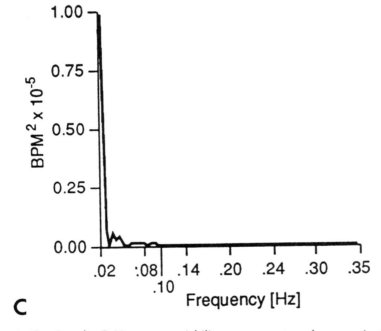

Figure 1. *(Continued)* **C.** Heart rate variability power spectrum from a patient with symptomatic systolic left ventricular dysfunction. Notice the overall decrease in the area under the curve (representing a decrease in total power) as well as the totally abolished high-frequency peak (representing decreased parasympathetically mediated responsiveness of the sinoatrial node). (A. Reproduced with permission from Reference 19; B. and C. reproduced with permission from Binkley PF, Nunziata E, Haas GJ, Nelson SD, Cody RJ: Parasympathetic withdrawal is an integral component of autonomic imbalance in congestive heart failure: demonstration in human subjects and verification in a paced canine model of ventricular failure. *J Am Coll Cardiol* 18:464–472, 1991.)

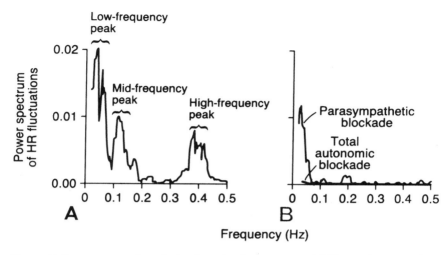

Figure 2. Power spectral analysis of canine heart rate variability under control (**A**) and selective autonomic blockade (**B**) conditions. (Reproduced with permission from Reference 5.)

the HRV power spectrum.[5-7,11-13,15] Of note, some studies have suggested that increased parasympathetic tone has a "protective effect" on ventricular myocardium, whereas increased sympathetic tone is proarrhythmic.[20-23] Although this is an oversimplification, observations on HRV made in patients after infarction and in those with congestive heart failure support these notions.[4,14,18,23,24]

Heart Rate Variability in Acute Myocardial Infarction

In the Multicenter Post-Infarction Program (MPIP), Kleiger et al[14] reported that decreased HRV (standard deviation of all normal RR intervals in an entire 24-hour ECG recording [SDNN] ≤ 15 milliseconds) was a significant risk stratifier of all causes of mortality independent of mean heart rate, ventricular ectopic activity, left ventricular function, and New York Heart Association class. Many other authors have corroborated the data from this study.[9,10,25,26] Bigger et al[9,10] reported the time course of recovery of HRV in patients after myocardial infarction and noted an acute decrease in HRV, followed by a statistically significant increase in HRV within 3 months. HRV then plateaued and remained unchanged for up to 12 months after myocardial infarction, at

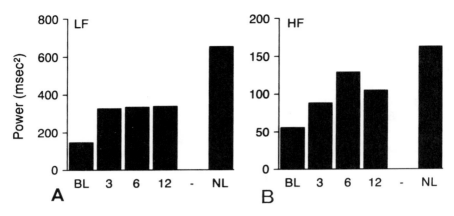

Figure 3. Time course of recovery in low-frequency (LF, **A**) and high-frequency (HF, **B**) power after myocardial infarction. Power is plotted at baseline (BL), 3, 6, and 12 months after myocardial infarction and for noninfarcted controls. NL = normal persons. See text for details. (Reproduced with permission from Reference 10.)

which point it was still statistically significantly below that of normal subjects (Figure 3).

HRV has also been investigated in the acute phase of myocardial infarction in relation to patency of the infarct-related artery, infarct location, life-threatening ventricular arrhythmias, and life-threatening congestive heart failure.[2,4,20,25,27–31] Zabel et al[2] reported changes in HRV with angiographically determined patency after thrombolysis in patients with acute myocardial infarction. In the first hour after the initiation of thrombolysis, the percentage of differences between adjacent normal RR intervals that were > 50 milliseconds computed over an entire 24-hour ECG recording (pNN50) was increased significantly in patients with successful reperfusion in comparison with those without successful reperfusion (12.6% ± 12.4% and 6.6% ± 7.3%, respectively, $P = 0.024$). Hermosillo et al[31] reported that patients with spontaneous or drug-induced reperfusion have increased high-frequency HRV in comparison with patients with closed infarct-related arteries. Also, patients with closed infarct-related arteries have reduced HRV and lower low-frequency and high-frequency power spectral density than healthy control subjects. Luria et al[30] reported a decrease in HRV during the first 24 hours after thrombolytic therapy for acute myocardial infarction in a group of 81 patients compared with 41 age-matched normal subjects. Of interest, in patients with anterior myocardial infarction, HRV diminished more rapidly than in those with inferior myocardial infarction. Also, patients with anterior myocardial infarction had significantly higher heart rates and decreased HRV than those with inferior infarcts. Pedretti et al,[28] in a group of 30 patients who received thrombolysis within 6 hours after the onset of symptoms, reported higher HRV in the time domain than in 21 patients with acute myocardial infarction who had contraindications to thrombolysis. As expected, the thrombolytic group had a lower incidence of arrhythmic events and was less likely to have inducible ventricular tachycardia on invasive electrophysiologic testing (P = 0.002). In patients with anterior myocardial infarction, the difference was more pronounced. SDNN equaled 118 ± 41 milliseconds for those receiving thrombolysis and 74 ± 24 milliseconds for those not receiving lytic therapy (P = 0.002). This difference in HRV was evident despite similar ejection fractions in the two groups (38% ± 6% and 36% ± 8% in the lytic and nonlytic groups, respectively). Despite these studies, an absolute value of HRV time- or frequency-domain variables or a percentage change in such variables has not been tested rigorously in a controlled, prospective manner to determine the predictive value of HRV in identifying the patency of an infarct-related artery.

In addition to its association with the patency of an infarct-related artery, HRV is a useful stratifier of early mortality after myocardial infarction.[25,27,32,33] Wolf et al[33] reported a 3.8-fold increase in relative risk for in-hospital death in patients with low RR interval variance after myocardial infarction. Vaishnav et al[27] reported time- and frequency-domain analysis of HRV and mortality in 226 consecutive patients with acute myocardial infarction. SDNN and low-frequency HRV measured within an average of 3.5 days after myocardial infarction were decreased significantly (P = 0.0003 and P = 0.0001, respectively) in nonsurvivors compared with survivors followed over an 8-month period after infarction. Casolo et al[25] also found that HRV measured 2 to 3 days after myocardial infarction was decreased in patients who died less than 20 days after hospital admission for acute myocardial infarction. In these high-risk patients, the 24-hour RR interval standard deviation was 31 ± 12 milliseconds, as compared with 60 ± 20 milliseconds for survivors (P < 0.001). Also, a value of 24-hour RR interval standard deviation less than 50 milliseconds was significantly associated with increased mortality, higher Killip class, and the use of diuretics or digitalis (P < 0.025, 0.004, 0.001, and 0.024, respectively).

In summary, HRV is a useful risk stratifier in the setting of acute myocardial infarction. Early mortality, heart failure, life-threatening ventricular arrhythmia, patency of the infarct-related artery, and infarct location are all associated with diminished HRV. However, although HRV has been reported by some authors to be predictive independently of infarct size and left ventricular function, it is still unclear whether prospective analysis of HRV in the setting of acute myocardial infarction would affect individual patient outcome.

Conclusion

In the setting of acute myocardial infarction, much has been learned from signal processing of the surface ECG. Spectral processing techniques have been applied to both beat-to-beat changes in heart period and beat-to-beat changes in QRST morphology. Both time-domain and frequency-domain analyses of HRV have revealed a marked diminution in HRV in patients with acute myocardial infarction. In general, HRV is decreased in patients with anterior myocardial infarction, particularly with anterior myocardial infarction versus inferior myocardial infarction. It is also decreased in patients with nonpatent infarct-related arteries versus patent infarct-related arteries, in nonsurvivors versus survivors of myocardial infarction, in Q-wave infarcts versus non-Q-wave infarcts,[25] and in patients who did not receive thrombolytic therapy for myocardial infarction versus those who did receive this treatment. Although these techniques are helpful in risk stratification of patients after myocardial infarction, it is unclear whether analysis of HRV in the setting of acute myocardial infarction would have a positive effect on treatment.

References

1. Krone RJ: The role of risk stratification in the early management of a myocardial infarction. *Ann Intern Med* 116:223–237, 1992.
2. Zabel M, Klingenheben T, Hohnloser SH: Changes in autonomic tone following thrombolytic therapy for acute myocardial infarction: assessment by analysis of heart rate variability. *J Cardiovasc Electrophysiol* 5:211–218, 1994.
3. Odemuyiwa O, Jordaan P, Malik M, et al: Autonomic correlates of late infarct artery patency after first myocardial infarction. *Am Heart J* 125:1597–1600, 1993.
4. Carter JE Jr, Childers RW: Torsades de pointes complicating acute myocardial infarction: the importance of autonomic dysfunction as assessed by heart rate variability. *Clin Cardiol* 15:769–772, 1992.
5. Akselrod S, Gordon D, Ubel FA, Shannon DC, Berger AC, Cohen RJ: Power spectrum analysis of heart rate fluctuation: a quantitative probe of beat-to-beat cardiovascular control. *Science* 213:220–222, 1981.
6. Saul JP, Rea RF, Eckberg DL, Berger RD, Cohen RJ: Heart rate and muscle sympathetic nerve variability during reflex changes of autonomic activity. *Am J Physiol* 258:H713-H721, 1990.
7. Saul JP: Beat-to-beat variations of heart rate reflect modulation of cardiac autonomic outflow. *News Physiol Sci* 5:32–37, 1990.
8. van Ravenswaaij-Arts CM, Kollee LA, Hopman JC, Stoelinga GB, van Geijn HP: Heart rate variability. *Ann Intern Med* 118:436–447, 1993.
9. Bigger JT Jr, Fleiss JL, Rolnitzky LM, Steinman RC: Stability over time of heart period variability in patients with previous myocardial infarction and ventricular arrhythmias. The CAPS and ESVEM investigators. *Am J Cardiol* 69:718–723, 1992.

10. Bigger JT Jr, Fleiss JL, Rolnitzky LM, Steinman RC, Schneider WJ: Time course of recovery of heart period variability after myocardial infarction. *J Am Coll Cardiol* 18:1643–1649, 1991.
11. Challis RE, Kitney RI: Biomedical signal processing (in four parts). Part 1. Time-domain methods. *Med Biol Eng Comput* 28:509–524, 1990.
12. Challis RE, Kitney RI: Biomedical signal processing (in four parts). Part 2. The frequency transforms and their interrelationships. *Med Biol Eng Comput* 29: 1–17, 1991.
13. Challis RE, Kitney RI: Biomedical signal processing (in four parts). Part 3. The power spectrum and coherence function. *Med Biol Eng Comput* 29:225–241, 1991.
14. Kleiger RE, Miller JP, Bigger JT Jr, Moss AJ: Decreased heart rate variability and its association with increased mortality after acute myocardial infarction. *Am J Cardiol* 59:256–262, 1987.
15. Kitney RI, Rompelman O (eds): *The Study of Heart-Rate Variability.* New York: Oxford University Press; 1980.
16. Berger RD, Akselrod S, Gordon D, Cohen RJ: An efficient algorithm for spectral analysis of heart rate variability. *IEEE Trans Biomed Eng* 33:900–904, 1986.
17. DeBoer RW, Karemaker JM, Strackee J: Comparing spectra of a series of point events particularly for heart rate variability data. *IEEE Trans Biomed Eng* BME-31;384–387, 1984.
18. Myers GA, Martin GJ, Magid NM, et al: Power spectral analysis of heart rate variability in sudden cardiac death: comparison to other methods. *IEEE Trans Biomed Eng* 33:1149–1156, 1986.
19. Pieper SJ, Hammill SC: Heart rate variability: technique and investigational applications in cardiovascular medicine. *Mayo Clin Proc* 70:955–964, 1995.
20. Valkama JO, Huikuri HV, Airaksinen KE, Linnaluoto MK, Takkunen JT: Changes in frequency domain measures of heart rate variability in relation to the onset of ventricular tachycardia in acute myocardial infarction. *Int J Cardiol* 38:177–182, 1993.
21. Lown B, Verrier RL: Neural activity and ventricular fibrillation. *N Engl J Med* 294:1165–1170, 1976.
22. Lombardi F, Verrier RL, Lown B: Relationship between sympathetic neural activity, coronary dynamics, and vulnerability to ventricular fibrillation during myocardial ischemia and reperfusion. *Am Heart J* 105:958–965, 1983.
23. McAreavey D, Neilson JM, Ewing DJ, Russell DC: Cardiac parasympathetic activity during the early hours of acute myocardial infarction. *Br Heart J* 62:165–170, 1989.
24. Surawicz B, Fisch C: Cardiac alternans: diverse mechanisms and clinical manifestations. *J Am Coll Cardiol* 20:483–499, 1992.
25. Casolo GC, Stroder P, Signorini C, et al: Heart rate variability during the acute phase of myocardial infarction. *Circulation* 85:2073–2079, 1992.
26. Farrell TG, Bashir Y, Cripps T, et al: Risk stratification for arrhythmic events in postinfarction patients based on heart rate variability, ambulatory electrocardiographic variables and the signal-averaged electrocardiogram. *J Am Coll Cardiol* 18:687–697, 1991.
27. Vaishnav S, Stevenson R, Marchant B, Lagi K, Ranjadayalan K, Timmis AD: Relation between heart rate variability early after acute myocardial infarction and long-term mortality. *Am J Cardiol* 73:653–657, 1994.
28. Pedretti RF, Colombo E, Sarzi Braga S, Caru B: Effect of thrombolysis on heart

rate variability and life-threatening ventricular arrhythmias in survivors of acute myocardial infarction. *J Am Coll Cardiol* 23:19–26, 1994.

29. Marchant B, Stevenson R, Vaishnav S, Ranjadayalan K, Timmis AD: Myocardial ischaemia and angina in the early post-infarction period: a comparison with patients with stable coronary artery disease. *Br Heart J* 70:438–442, 1993.

30. Luria MH, Sapoznikov D, Gilon D, et al: Early heart rate variability alterations after acute myocardial infarction. *Am Heart J* 125:676–681, 1993.

31. Hermosillo AG, Dorado M, Casanova JM, et al: Influence of infarct-related artery patency on the indexes of parasympathetic activity and prevalence of late potentials in survivors of acute myocardial infarction. *J Am Coll Cardiol* 22:695–706, 1993.

32. Pipilis A, Flather M, Ormerod O, Sleight P: Heart rate variability in acute myocardial infarction and its association with infarct site and clinical course. *Am J Cardiol* 67:1137–1139, 1991.

33. Wolf MM, Varigos GA, Hunt D, Sloman JG: Sinus arrhythmia in acute myocardial infarction. *Med J Aust* 2:52–53, 1978.

5

Electrical Alternans

Stephen J. Pieper, MD

Alternating amplitude from beat-to-beat of portions of the electrocardiogram (ECG) has been observed on many occasions. The ECG manifestations of electrical alternans were divided into five categories by Lepeschkin in 1950[1]: 1) alternating conduction delay; 2) primary alterations in ST-segment morphology; 3) T-wave alternans; 4) electrical alternans secondary to mechanical alternans; and 5) a combination of 1 to 4. The following discussion focuses on alternans during myocardial ischemia, mainly as related to alternans in ST-T segments. Alternans associated with conduction delay and mechanical alternans are mentioned briefly. Electrical alternans associated with supraventricular tachycardias and various types of ventricular tachycardias have been well described, but are not particularly manifestations of myocardial ischemia or injury.[2]

Alternans of conduction is manifested as altered duration or morphology of P waves, PR intervals, or the QRS complex (such as alternation of right or left bundle branch block).[2] These changes occur most commonly with rapid heart rates, but have been recorded at normal heart rates as well.[2] Myocardial ischemia can be a precipitating factor for conduction alternans. However, most descriptions of clinical electrical alternans associated with myocardial ischemia are manifested as ST-T-wave alternans.[2-10] An example of ST-T-wave alternans is given in Figure 1.

The mechanism of ST-T-wave alternans during ischemia is thought to be related to electrical inhomogeneities within the ischemic myocardium, as well as between the ischemic myocardium and the normal myocardium.[2,9,11-13] Autonomic stimulation, intracellular calcium cycling, and alteration in potassium and sodium handling in ischemic

From: Clements, IP (ed). *The Electrocardiogram in Acute Myocardial Infarction.* Armonk, NY: Futura Publishing Company, Inc. © Mayo Foundation 1998.

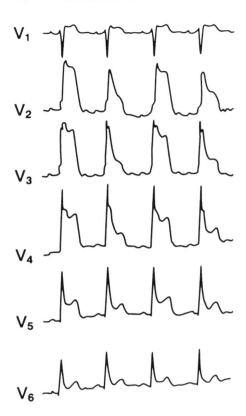

Figure 1. Precordial surface electrocardiogram (ECG) leads from a patient with acute myocardial injury and associated ECG alternans. Alternation in the ST-T-wave segment amplitude can readily be seen in leads V_2 to V_5. (Reproduced with permission from Reference 15.)

myocardium have all been implicated in the genesis of ST-T-wave alternans, particularly as these factors relate to action-potential morphology, dispersion of refractiveness, and recovery of excitability.[14-17] Correlations between ischemia-induced electrical alternans at the cellular level and alternans in ST segments have been made.[4,15,18] Most commonly, alternation is seen in the magnitude of ST-segment elevation or T-wave morphology.[2,4,15] Several groups of investigators have reported a significant association between the occurrence of visible T-wave alternans and ventricular arrhythmias in patients with variant angina.[19-22] Turitto and El-Sherif[22] reported a correlation among alternans, arrhythmias, and coronary occlusion in patients with Prinzmetal's angina.

Although these changes can be seen grossly on the surface ECG, they are rare. Spectral analysis has been used to provide a more sensitive and quantitative technique for relating electrical alternans to myocardial vulnerability and impending ventricular fibrillation.[3,4,23-28] Nearing and Verrier[4] reported a statistically significant increase in "alternans level" in mongrel dogs that fibrillated shortly after occlusion of the left anterior descending coronary artery.

In the clinical setting, Rosenbaum et al[29] used a spectral technique to test the hypothesis that "electrical alternans is a marker of vulnerability to ventricular arrhythmias" in patients referred for electrophysiologic study. Spectral analysis with right atrial pacing at a rate of 100/minute demonstrated subtle alternans of the T-wave magnitude not visible on the surface ECG (Figure 2). Electrical alternans was a significant predictor of inducibility of ventricular arrhythmias during the electrophysiologic study. In that study, the presence of organic heart disease, history of myocardial infarction, and decreased left ventricular ejection fraction did not discriminate between patients with negative findings

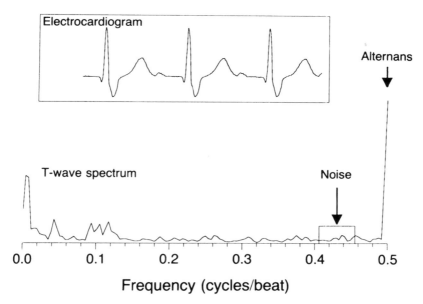

Figure 2. Representative example of the use of a computer algorithm to detect low-level beat-to-beat oscillations of the surface morphology of the electrocardiogram (ECG). One hundred twenty-eight consecutive ECG complexes recorded from three orthogonal leads were used to generate the representation of beat-to-beat oscillations in the amplitude of the ECG. The **inset** shows a segment of one ECG lead (X) from which the T-wave power spectrum was derived. T-wave alternans is measured from the amplitude of the peak of the power spectrum at the alternans frequency (0.5 cycle per beat) and is compared with the amplitude of the power spectrum measured in a predetermined noise window. Despite the absence of any visible beat-to-beat alternation of T-wave amplitude (**inset**), a clear peak is evident at the alternans frequency that cannot be attributed to noise. (Reproduced with permission from Reference 29.)

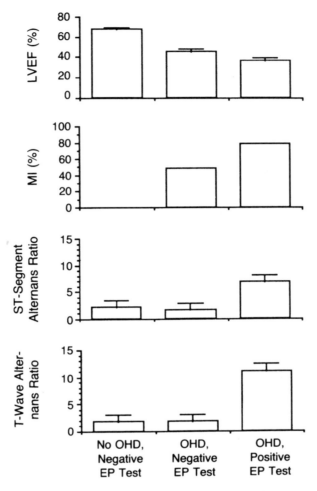

Figure 3. Left ventricular ejection fraction (LVEF), percentage of patients with a history of myocardial infarction (MI), and alternans ratios in the ST segment and T wave in subgroups of patients. Included in this analysis were 20 patients without organic heart disease (OHD), all of whom had negative electrophysiologic (EP) tests; 31 patients with OHD in whom ventricular arrhythmias could not be elicited by programmed stimulation during EP testing; and 32 patients with OHD who had positive EP tests. As expected, patients with OHD had a lower LVEF and a higher prevalence of MI. The presence of OHD, by itself, was not associated with increased T-wave or ST-segment alternans ratios (i.e., alternans ratios > 2.5). Alternans ratios were significantly elevated only in patients who were susceptible to inducible ventricular arrhythmias. Therefore, repolarization alternans was a marker of electrical and not mechanical cardiac dysfunction. The values shown are means ± SE. (Reproduced with permission from Reference 29.)

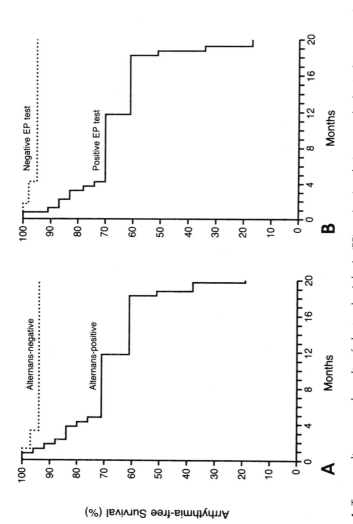

Figure 4. T-wave alternans and results of electrophysiologic (EP) testing in relation to arrhythmia-free survival among 66 patients. **A.** Arrhythmia-free survival according to Kaplan-Meier life-table analysis is compared in patients with T-wave alternans (alternans ratio, > 3.0) and without it (ratio, ≤ 3.0). Note that the presence of T-wave alternans is a strong predictor of reduced arrhythmia-free survival. **B.** Arrhythmia-free survival among patients with positive EP tests is compared with that among patients in whom ventricular arrhythmias were not induced on EP testing (negative EP test). The predictive value of EP testing and T-wave alternans is essentially the same in these plots. (Reproduced with permission from Reference 29.)

on electrophysiologic tests and those with positive findings (Figure 3). Also, the levels of T-wave alternans were significantly greater in patients who had arrhythmic events over a 20-month follow-up period (relative risk = 9.0) and appeared equal to the predictive ability of electrophysiologic testing (Figure 4). In a subgroup of 45 patients not receiving antiarrhythmic drugs, arrhythmic-free survival was 44% and 94% for alternans-positive versus alternans-negative patients, respectively. Other authors have presented evidence that electrical alternans occurs regionally before it is seen on the surface ECG.[7,30] Salerno et al[7] reported that acute myocardial ischemia produced impaired conduction and repolarization dispersion that correlated with T-wave alternans and arrhythmogenesis in humans. Sutton et al[30] reported alternans in action-potential recordings from 14 of 36 patients undergoing cardiopulmonary bypass surgery. Monophasic action-potential recordings from the left ventricular epicardium revealed action-potential alternans with short duration (> 90 seconds) occlusions of coronary artery grafts. Because this phenomenon was localized to small areas of the myocardium and none of the patients manifested alternans on their surface ECGs, the authors suggested that "the clinical ECG may be silent to this potential prearrhythmic situation."

Conclusions

In summary, the ECG manifestations of ischemic electrical alternans are most commonly seen in alternation in ST-segment elevation magnitude or alternation of T-wave morphology (or both). These changes correlate well with models of ischemic-induced changes in refractoriness and in action-potential morphology during repolarization. These changes also are enhanced by alterations in autonomic tone that are associated with myocardial ischemia. Although the surface ECG may show visible alternans of the ST-T segment, it is not a sensitive technique. Signal-processing techniques such as spectral analysis and complex demodulation have been applied to the surface ECG in the postinfarction and acute coronary occlusive settings in an attempt to quantitate subtle changes in the surface ECG ST-T segment. Such analyses have proven beneficial in risk stratification for life-threatening arrhythmic events in selected patient groups. However, the benefit and applicability of these techniques on a routine clinical basis have not been documented.

References

1. Lepeschkin E: Electrocardiographic observations on mechanism of electrical alternans of heart. *Cardiologia* 16:278–287, 1950.

2. Surawicz B, Fisch C: Cardiac alternans: diverse mechanisms and clinical manifestations. *J Am Coll Cardiol* 20:483–499, 1992.

3. Verrier RL, Nearing BD: Electrophysiologic basis for T wave alternans as an index of vulnerability to ventricular fibrillation. *J Cardiovasc Electrophysiol* 5: 445–461, 1994.

4. Nearing BD, Verrier RL: T-wave alternans magnitude but not ST-segment changes correlate with spontaneous ventricular tachycardia and fibrillation during coronary artery occlusion and reperfusion in canines (abstr). *Circulation* 88: I-627, 1993.

5. Elharrar V, Zipes DP: Cardiac electrophysiologic alterations during myocardial ischemia. *Am J Physiol* 233:H329-H345, 1997.

6. Joyal M, Feldman RL, Pepine CJ: ST-segment alternans during percutaneous transluminal coronary angioplasty. *Am J Cardiol* 54:915–916, 1984.

7. Salerno JA, Previtali M, Panciroli C, et al: Ventricular arrhythmias during acute myocardial ischaemia in man. The role and significance of R-ST-T alternans and the prevention of ischaemic sudden death by medical treatment. *Eur Heart J* 7(suppl A):63–75, 1986.

8. Hashimoto H, Suzuki K, Miyake S, Nakashima M: Effects of calcium antagonists on the electrical alternans of the ST segment and on associated mechanical alternans during acute coronary occlusion in dogs. *Circulation* 68:667–672, 1983.

9. Hellerstein HK, Liebow IM: Electrical alternation in experimental coronary artery occlusion. *Am J Physiol* 160:366–374, 1950.

10. Puletti M, Curione M, Righetti G, Jacobellis G: Alternans of the ST segment and T wave in acute myocardial infarction. *J Electrocardiol* 13:297–300, 1980.

11. Corbalan R, Verrier RL, Lown B: Differing mechanisms for ventricular vulnerability during coronary artery occlusion and release. *Am Heart J* 92:223–230, 1976.

12. Kleber AG, Janse MJ, van Capelle FJ, Durrer D: Mechanism and time course of S-T and T-Q segment changes during acute regional myocardial ischemia in the pig heart determined by extracellular and intracellular recordings. *Circ Res* 42: 603–613, 1978.

13. Abe S, Nagamoto Y, Fukuchi Y, Hayakawa T, Kuroiwa A: Relationship of alternans of monophasic action potential and conduction delay inside the ischemic border zone to serious ventricular arrhythmia during acute myocardial ischemia in dogs. *Am Heart J* 117:1223–1233, 1989.

14. Lown B, Verrier RL: Neural activity and ventricular fibrillation. *N Engl J Med* 294:1165–1170, 1976.

15. Cinca J, Janse MJ, Morena H, Candell J, Valle V, Durrer D: Mechanism and time course of the early electrical changes during acute coronary artery occlusion. An attempt to correlate the early ECG changes in man to the cellular electrophysiology in the pig. *Chest* 77:499–505, 1980.

16. Levy MN: Role of calcium in arrhythmogenesis. *Circulation* 80(suppl IV):IV23-IV30, 1989.

17. Billman GE: The antiarrhythmic and antifibrillatory effects of calcium antagonists. *J Cardiovasc Pharmacol* 18(suppl 10):S107-S117, 1991.

18. Downar E, Janse MJ, Durrer D: The effect of acute coronary artery occlusion on subepicardial transmembrane potentials in the intact porcine heart. *Circulation* 56:217–224, 1977.

19. Kleinfeld MJ, Rozanski JJ: Alternans of the ST segment in Prinzmetal's angina. *Circulation* 55:574–577, 1977.

20. Rozanski JJ, Kleinfeld M: Alternans of the ST segment of T wave. A sign of electrical instability in Prinzmetal's angina. *Pacing Clin Electrophysiol* 5: 359–365, 1982.
21. Cheng TC: Electrical alternans. An association with coronary artery spasm. *Arch Intern Med* 143:1052–1053, 1983.
22. Turitto G, El-Sherif N: Alternans of the ST segment in variant angina. Incidence, time course and relation to ventricular arrhythmias during ambulatory electrocardiographic recording. *Chest* 93:587–591, 1988.
23. Nearing BD, Verrier RL: Personal computer system for tracking cardiac vulnerability by complex demodulation of the T wave. *J Appl Physiol* 74:2606–2612, 1993.
24. Gilchrist IC: Prevalence and significance of ST-segment alternans during coronary angioplasty. *Am J Cardiol* 68:1534–1535, 1991.
25. Adam DR, Smith JM, Akselrod S, Nyberg S, Powell AO, Cohen RJ: Fluctuations in T-wave morphology and susceptibility to ventricular fibrillation. *J Electrocardiol* 17:209–218, 1984.
26. Konta T, Ikeda K, Yamaki M, et al: Significance of discordant ST alternans in ventricular fibrillation. *Circulation* 82:2185–2189, 1990.
27. Raeder EA, Rosenbaum DS, Bhasin R, Cohen RJ: Alternating morphology of the QRST complex preceding sudden death (letter). *N Engl J Med* 326:271–272, 1992.
28. Nearing BD, Huang AH, Verrier RL: Dynamic tracking of cardiac vulnerability by complex demodulation of the T wave. *Science* 252:437–440, 1991.
29. Rosenbaum DS, Jackson LE, Smith JM, Garan H, Ruskin JN, Cohen RJ: Electrical alternans and vulnerability to ventricular arrhythmias. *N Engl J Med* 330: 235–241, 1994.
30. Sutton PM, Taggart P, Lab M, Runnalls ME, O'Brien W, Treasure T: Alternans of epicardial repolarization as a localized phenomenon in man. *Eur Heart J* 12: 70–78, 1991.

6

Signal-Averaged Electrocardiogram and Acute Myocardial Infarction

Ian P. Clements, MD

The terminal portion of the QRS complex contains information predictive of electrical instability.[1-3] Analysis of this portion of the electrocardiogram (ECG) is performed on a signal-averaged ECG (SA-ECG). The SA-ECG has been used in cases of acute and chronic myocardial infarction as a predictor of life-threatening ventricular arrhythmias.[4] Of note is that reperfusion in the setting of acute infarction decreases the frequency of abnormalities found on the SA-ECG after infarction,[5] and it has been suggested that this change represents improved electrical stability with reperfusion after infarction and contributes, in part, to the decreased mortality associated with reperfusion after infarction.

Recording the SA-ECG

The recording of the SA-ECG requires attention to detail.[6] The late potentials are low amplitude (usually $< 10~\mu V$) and can be masked by background noise. Thus, special adaptations of the ECG recording device are necessary to decrease electromagnetic interference. It is important to obtain a stable and good skin-electrode interface, and the patient should be comfortable and relaxed during the recording.

Because of the low noise-to-signal ratio of the late potential, the signal-averaging process, by recording 100 to 400 sinus beats, reduces

From: Clements, IP (ed). *The Electrocardiogram in Acute Myocardial Infarction.* Armonk, NY: Futura Publishing Company, Inc. © Mayo Foundation 1998.

the noise level of the signal by the square root of the number of cycles recorded.

Other variables are important in SA-ECG recording. It is important that the standard QRS complex be recorded; thus, recording devices use a template-recognition program to reject nonstandard QRS complexes, such as ventricular ectopic beats. The QRS complexes must be aligned carefully.

The SA-ECG is lead-dependent, but it is usually recorded from bi-polar X, Y, and Z leads, using American Heart Association criteria.[7] High-pass filtering is used to further reduce noise.

Thus, the recording of the SA-ECG involves careful attention to the recording method, because variation in the recording method can alter the measurement of the SA-ECG variables.

SA-ECG Variables

Simson[8] defined three variables from the SA-ECG. The onset and offset of the QRS complex are defined and, thus, the first variable, the duration of the QRS complex, is measured. The duration of the late potential less than 40 μV at the end of the QRS complex is the second variable that is measured. The root-mean-square of the voltage during the last 40 milliseconds of the QRS is the third variable recorded from the SA-ECG (Figure 1). Table 1 provides the normal values for these variables, as obtained by several investigators using high-pass filters.

Late Potentials and Acute Myocardial Infarction

A number of studies have analyzed the incidence and evolution of late potentials after the onset of acute myocardial infarction.[4,16,17] It is of note that late potentials are more frequent in patients with an inferior than in those with an anterior myocardial infarction.[16] This is a consequence of the later activation of the basal portions of the myocardium. Thus, if abnormalities are present in the basal myocardium, they are more likely to be seen on the later portion of the QRS complex, which explains the greater likelihood of seeing late potentials in patients with an inferior infarction (Figures 2A and 2B).

Late potentials can be detected in the initial hours after myocardial infarction. McGuire et al[18] noted a 32% incidence of late potentials at 12.4 ± 6.6 hours after the onset of symptoms of infarction (Figure 3). The incidence increased to 52% by the time of dismissal from the hospital. In that study, 8 of the 21 patients with late potentials on the initial recording developed early ventricular tachycardia or fibrillation, in contrast with 2 of 35 patients without late potentials. However, other inves-

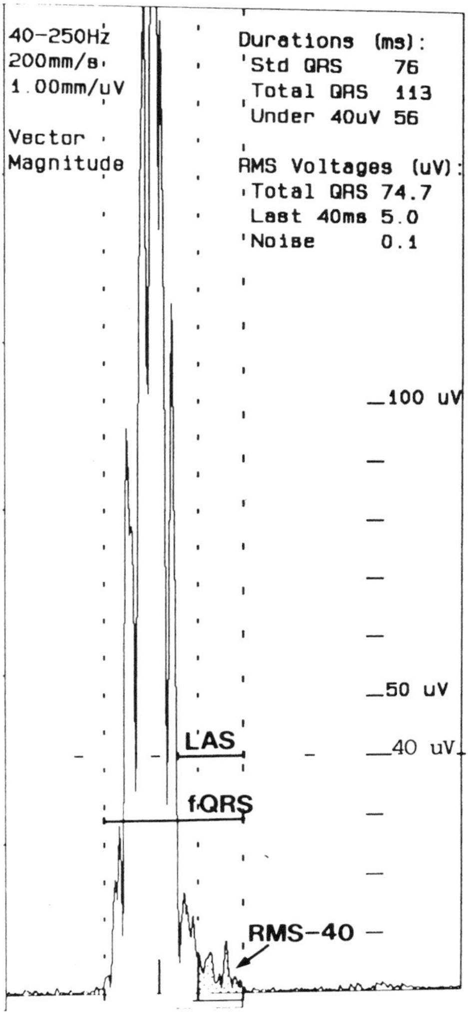

Figure 1. Example of an abnormal signal-averaged electrocardiogram showing the three commonly measured variables: the duration of the QRS complex (fQRS), the duration of the low-amplitude signal (< 40 μV) (LAS), and the root-mean-square (RMS) of the last 40 milliseconds of the QRS. (Reproduced with permission from Reference 6.)

tigators have not noted a similar ominous significance for early late potentials after myocardial infarction.[19]

The presence or absence of late potentials evolve in the days after myocardial infarction. El-Sherif et al[19] demonstrated that the incidence of late potentials was 17%, 25%, and 18% from days 0 to 5, 6 to 30, and 31 to 60, respectively, up to the onset of acute infarction. They also found that the presence of late potentials between days 6 and 30 was the factor most predictive of an arrhythmic event. Of 12 patients with

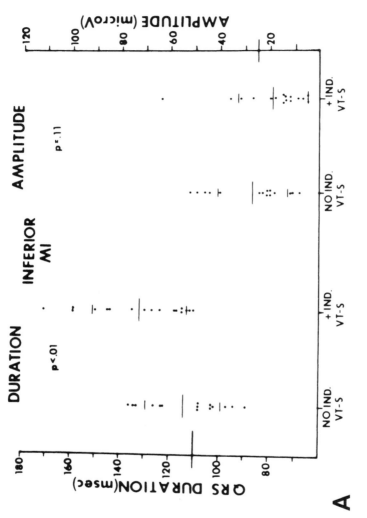

Figure 2. The duration of the QRS complex and the amplitude of the last 40 milliseconds of the complex in, **A**, patients with an inferior myocardial infarction (MI) and, **B**, those with an anterior MI. QRS duration greater than 110 milliseconds was considered highly sensitive for detecting the patients with an inferior MI likely to have

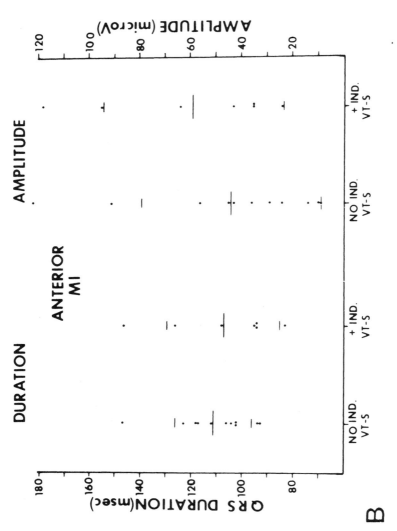

Figure 2. *(Continued)* inducible sustained ventricular tachycardia. The signal-averaged ECG was not helpful in detecting inducible sustained ventricular tachycardia in patients with an anterior MI. (Reproduced with permission from Reference 16.)

Table 1
Normal Values of Signal-Averaged Electrocardiographic Variables

Author	No. of Subjects	Age,* yr	QRS,* ms	FP, %	LAS,* ms	FP, %	RMS-40,* μV	FP, %
25-Hz high pass filter								
Denes et al[9]	42	34 ± 2	95.9 ± 1.4 <120	0	23.3 ± 1.1 ≤30	21	67.1 ± 5.2 >25	4
Gomes et al[10]	25	34 ± 10	94 ± 10 <114	—	20 ± 6 <32	—	117 ± 103 >25	—
Flowers and Wylds[11]	67	28 ± 9	93.8 ± 1.6	—	20 ± 0.7	—	87.4 ± 7.7	4
Caref et al[12]	100	31 ± 9	94.4 ± 10.1 ≤115	—	18.8 ± 6.8 ≤32	—	96.9 ± 60.3 ≥25	—
Poll et al[13]	55	36 ± 11	95.9 ± 91	0	—	—	53.7 ± 25.2	7
Freedman et al[14]	19	30 ± 4	—	—	—	—	87.5	0
Danford et al[15]	32	25 ± 4	97.3 ± 9.4 M < 117 F < 102	—	20.4 ± 7.2 <35	—	88.9 ± 54.9 >20	—
40-Hz high pass filter								
Denes et al[9]	42	34 ± 2	93.7 ± 1.4 <120	0	29.5 ± 1.1 <39	10	41.6 ± 3.5 >20	10
Gomes et al[10]	25	34 ± 10	92 ± 11 <114	—	26 ± 6 <38	—	81 ± 65 >20	—
Caref et al[12]	100	31 ± 9	92.4 ± 9.5 ≤111	—	24.1 ± 7.3 ≤39	—	58.4 ± 38.7 ≥16	—
Danford et al[15]	27	28 ± 4	94.2 ± 12.6	—	24.9 ± 11.0	—	58.0 ± 32.6	—
80-Hz high-pass filter								
Gomes et al[10]	25	34 ± 10	87 ± 10 <107	—	30 ± 6 <42	—	47 ± 54 >17	—
Caref et al[12]	100	31 ± 10	87.9 ± 9.0 ≤106	—	32.2 ± 8.7 <50	—	29.0 ± 15.7 ≥9	—

FP = false positives; LAS = low-amplitude signal duration; QRS = filtered QRS duration; RMS-40 = root-mean-square amplitude of last 40 ms of vector magnitude.
* Values are mean ± SD.
(Reproduced with permission from Reference 6.)

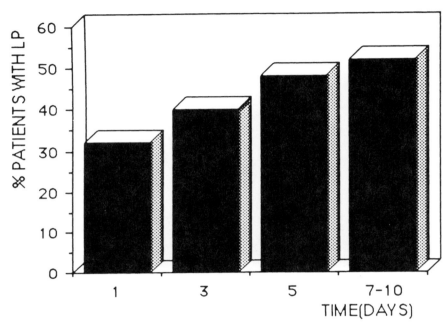

Figure 3. The prevalence of late potentials (LP) increases from day 1 through day 7 to 10 after myocardial infarction. (Reproduced with permission from Reference 18.)

ventricular tachycardia or fibrillation during the first year after infarction, 9 had the presence of late potentials on the SA-ECG. Most of the events occurred within 60 days after the onset of the infarct (Figure 4).

Influence of Thrombolysis and Patent Infarct-Related Artery

After thrombolysis, the development of late potentials is limited.[5] Thrombolysis appears to reduce the development of late potentials 2 days after the onset of infarction. In patients receiving conventional therapy, the incidence of late potentials increased from 12% to 23% after 2 days. This increase was not seen in patients receiving thrombolysis.[20]

It is of note that late potentials failed to develop after thrombolysis in patients with patent infarct-related arteries.[5] The GISSI-2 study demonstrated decreased incidence in late potentials in patients receiving thrombolysis (17%) in comparison with those receiving conventional treatment (29%).[21] Lange et al[22] noted a 40% incidence of late potentials

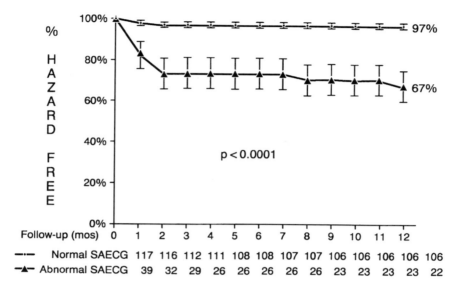

Follow-up (mos)	0	1	2	3	4	5	6	7	8	9	10	11	12
–·– Normal SAECG	117	116	112	111	108	108	107	107	106	106	106	106	106
–▲– Abnormal SAECG	39	32	29	26	26	26	26	26	23	23	23	23	22

Figure 4. Hazard curves comparing probability of remaining free of arrhythmic events in patients with normal and abnormal signal-averaged ECG (SA-ECG). Data presented as mean ± SEM. (Reproduced with permission from Reference 19.)

in patients with occluded infarct-related arteries, in comparison with 8% in patients with patent infarct-related arteries. Patients who underwent rescue angioplasty after thrombolysis continued to show a high incidence of abnormal SA-ECGs.

Thus, it has been postulated that some of the benefit of thrombolysis is related to the decreased incidence of late potentials and the lessening of the risk of life-threatening ventricular arrhythmias. Thrombolytic therapy administered 6 to 24 hours after the onset of acute infarction also reduced the frequency of abnormal SA-ECGs.[23] The sensitivity and specificity of the SA-ECG change after thrombolysis was not sufficient to allow detection of reperfusion.[24]

SA-ECG and Prognosis After Myocardial Infarction

The SA-ECG has been used to predict prognosis after myocardial infarction. The SA-ECG has been used either alone or in conjunction with an assessment of left ventricular function.

The presence of an abnormal signal-averaged ECG does suggest an increased risk of sudden death or ventricular tachydysrhythmia (Table

Table 2
Ability of SA-ECG to Predict Arrhythmic Events After Myocardial Infarction

Study	No. of Patients	F/U, mo	HPF, Hz	SA-ECG Variable	Abnormal SA-ECG, %	AE	No. of AE	Events Predicted	Sens, %	Spec, %	+Pred, %	−Pred, %
El-Sherif et al[19]	156	12	25	1 of 2: RMS ≤ 25, QRS ≥ 120	25	SCD, VT, VT-VF	4, 3, 5	All AE	75	79	23	97
Breithardt and Borggrefe[25]	511	18	100	Visual LP > 10 ms	38	SCD, VT	16, 14	SCD, VT	50, 79	62, 63	4, 6	87, 99
Subset[25]	222	—	—	Visual LP > 10 ms		VT	11	VT	—	—	9	—
von Leitner et al[26]	518	10	100	Visual LP > 10 ms	21	CD, SCD	8, 4	CD, SCD	57, 50	80, 79	7.3, 3.6	98.5, 99.1
Denniss et al[27]	306	12	0.05	VAT > 140 ms	26	SCD, VT-VF	12, 15	All AE	65	77	19	96
Kuchar et al[28]	210	14	40	Either: RMS-40 < 20 μV, QRS > 120 ms	39	SCD, VT	8, 7	All AE	93	65	17	99
Gomes et al[29]	102	12	40	One of: RMS-40 < 20 μV, LAS > 38 ms, QRS > 114 ms	44	SCD, VT, VT-VF	5, 7, 3	All AE	87	63	29	96.5
Cripps et al[30]	159	12	25	1 of 3: RMS < 25, LAS ≥ 25, QRS > 120	24	SCD, VT	5, 6	All AE	91	81	26	99
Verzoni et al[31]	220	8	40	2 of 3: RMS ≤ 20, LAS ≥ 40, QRS ≥ 120	28	SCD, VT	3, 3	All AE	83	73	8	99

AE = arrhythmic events; CD = cardiac death; F/U = follow-up; HPF = high-pass filter (corner frequency); LP = late potential; +Pred = positive predictive value; −Pred = negative predictive value; SA-ECG = signal-averaged ECG; SCD = sudden cardiac death; Sens = sensitivity; Spec = specificity; VAT = ventricular activation time; VF = ventricular fibrillation; VT = ventricular tachycardia.
(Reproduced with permission from Reference 6.)

2). Patients with an abnormal SA-ECG have a 4% to 29% incidence of such events over 1 year of follow-up, as compared with a 0.8% to 4.3% event rate in patients with a normal SA-ECG. El-Sherif et al[19] and Gomes et al[32] demonstrated that decreased left ventricular function (ejection fraction ≤ 40%) and an abnormal SA-ECG were independent predictors of sudden death and ventricular tachycardia (Figure 5). Gomes et al[29] also identified a subgroup of patients with a high risk of sudden death or ventricular tachycardia after myocardial infarction with the combination of abnormal SA-ECG, left ventricular ejection fraction ≥ 41%, and high-grade ectopy. Such patients had a 50% risk of events, but in the absence of these variables no events occurred. When two of the high-risk markers were present, the event rate was 34% to 37%, and when

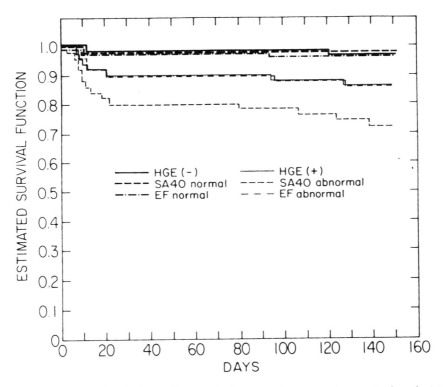

Figure 5. Estimated arrhythmia-free survival curves (Cox regression survival analysis) for 115 patients. The curves were plotted for the presence (+) or absence (-) of high-grade ectopy (HGE), abnormal signal-averaged ECG (SA40, 40-Hz high-grade filtering), or abnormal ejection fraction (EF) (EF < 40%). (Reproduced with permission from Reference 32.)

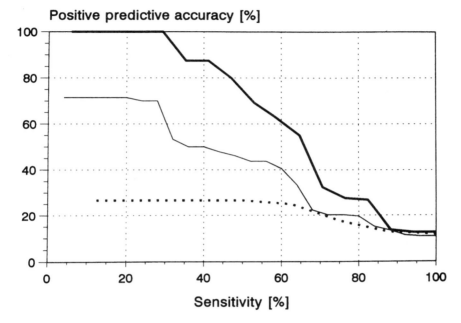

Positive predictive accuracy [%]

Figure 6. Positive predictive accuracy (y-axis) for arrhythmia events using the signal-averaged ECG. The positive predictive accuracy is much greater in patients not receiving thrombolysis (**thick line**) than in those receiving thrombolysis (**dotted line**). **Fine line** = positive predictive value for the whole population. (Reproduced with permission from Reference 33.)

two of these markers were absent, the rate was zero to 6%.[28,29] Studies have demonstrated that SA-ECG is superior to 24-hour monitoring in determining the risk of serious arrhythmias after myocardial infarction.[28,29]

An abnormal SA-ECG in patients who received thrombolysis was three times less predictive[33] of future events than it was in those who did not receive thrombolysis (Figure 6).

Summary

The SA-ECG can be used to predict arrhythmic events after myocardial infarction, and it is particularly useful in combination with an assessment of left ventricular function. Thrombolysis decreases the incidence of late potentials, particularly when associated with a patent infarct-related artery.[34]

References

1. Breithardt G, Becker R, Seipel L, Abendroth RR, Ostermeyer J: Noninvasive detection of late potentials in a man — a new marker for ventricular tachycardia. *Eur Heart J* 2:1–11, 1981.
2. Simson M, Horowitz L, Josephson M, Moore EN, Kastor J: A marker for ventricular tachycardia after myocardial infarction (abstr). *Circulation* 62(suppl 3):III-262, 1980.
3. Rozanski JJ, Mortara D, Myerburg RJ, Castellanos A: Body surface detection of delayed depolarizations in patients with recurrent ventricular tachycardia and left ventricular aneurysm. *Circulation* 63:1172–1178, 1981.
4. Breithardt G, Schwartzmaier J, Borggrefe M, Haerten K, Seipel L: Prognostic significance of late ventricular potentials after acute myocardial infarction. *Eur Heart J* 4:487–495, 1983.
5. Gang ES, Lew AS, Hong M, Wang FZ, Siebert CA, Peter T: Decreased incidence of ventricular late potentials after successful thrombolytic therapy for acute myocardial infarction. *N Engl J Med* 321:712–716, 1989.
6. Dunbar DN, Denes P: Operational aspects of signal-averaged electrocardiography. *Prog Cardiovasc Dis* 35:329–348, 1993.
7. Breithardt G, Cain ME, El-Sherif N, et al: Standards for analysis of ventricular late potentials using high-resolution or signal-averaged electrocardiography. A statement by a Task Force Committee of the European Society of Cardiology, the American Heart Association, and the American College of Cardiology. *Circulation* 83:1481–1488, 1991.
8. Simson MB: Use of signals in the terminal QRS complex to identify patients with ventricular tachycardia after myocardial infarction. *Circulation* 64:235–242, 1981.
9. Denes P, Santarelli P, Hauser RG, Uretz EF: Quantitative analysis of the high-frequency components of the terminal portion of the body surface QRS in normal subjects and in patients with ventricular tachycardia. *Circulation* 67:1129–1138, 1983.
10. Gomes JA, Winters SL, Stewart D, Targonski A, Barreca P: Optimal bandpass filters for time-domain analysis of the signal-averaged electrocardiogram. *Am J Cardiol* 60:1290–1298, 1987.
11. Flowers NC, Wylds AC: Ventricular late potentials in normal subjects. *Herz* 13: 160–168, 1988.
12. Caref EB, Turitto G, Ibrahim BB, Henkin R, El-Sherif N: Role of bandpass filters in optimizing the value of the signal-averaged electrocardiogram as a predictor of the results of programmed stimulation. *Am J Cardiol* 64:16–26, 1989.
13. Poll DS, Marchlinski FE, Falcone RA, Josephson ME, Simson MB: Abnormal signal-averaged electrocardiograms in patients with nonischemic congestive cardiomyopathy: relationship to sustained ventricular tachyarrhythmias. *Circulation* 72:1308–1313, 1985.
14. Freedman RA, Gillis AM, Keren A, Soderholm-Difatte V, Mason JW: Signal-averaged electrocardiographic late potentials in patients with ventricular fibrillation or ventricular tachycardia: correlation with clinical arrhythmia and electrophysiologic study. *Am J Cardiol* 55:1350–1353, 1985.
15. Danford DA, Stelling JA, Kugler JD, et al: Signal-averaged electrocardiography of the terminal QRS in healthy young adults. *Pacing Clin Electrophysiol* 12: 1712–1716, 1989.

16. Buxton AE, Britton N, Simson MB: Application of the signal-averaged electrocardiogram in patients with nonsustained ventricular tachycardia after myocardial infarction: implications for prediction of sudden cardiac death risk. *J Electrocardiol* 21(suppl):S-40-S-45, 1988.

17. Grimm M, Billhardt RA, Mayerhofer KE, Denes P: Prognostic significance of signal-averaged ECGs during acute myocardial infarction: a preliminary report. *J Electrocardiol* 21:283–288, 1988.

18. McGuire M, Kuchar D, Ganis J, Sammel N, Thorburn C: Natural history of late potentials in the first ten days after acute myocardial infarction and relation to early ventricular arrhythmias. *Am J Cardiol* 61:1187–1190, 1988.

19. El-Sherif N, Ursell SN, Bekheit S, et al: Prognostic significance of the signal-averaged ECG depends on the time of recording in the postinfarction period. *Am Heart J* 118:256–264, 1989.

20. Eldar M, Leor J, Hod H, et al: Effect of thrombolysis on the evolution of late potentials within 10 days of infarction. *Br Heart J* 63:273–276, 1990.

21. Riccio E, Cesaro F, Perotta R, Romano S, Correnle E, Corsini G: Early thrombolysis, reperfusion arrhythmias and late potentials in acute myocardial infarction. *New Trends in Arrhythmias* 6:157–161, 1990.

22. Lange RA, Cigarroa RG, Wells PJ, Kremers MS, Hills LD: Influence of anterograde flow in the infarct artery on the incidence of late potentials after acute myocardial infarction. *Am J Cardiol* 65:554–558, 1990.

23. Steinberg JS, Hochman JS, Morgan CD, LATE Ancillary Study Investigators, et al: Effects of thrombolytic therapy administered 6 to 24 hours after myocardial infarction on the signal-averaged ECG. Results of a multicenter randomized trial. *Circulation* 90:746–752, 1994.

24. Tranchesi B Jr, Verstraete M, Van de Werf F, et al: Usefulness of high-frequency analysis of signal-averaged surface electrocardiograms in acute myocardial infarction before and after coronary thrombolysis for assessing coronary reperfusion. *Am J Cardiol* 66:1196–1198, 1990.

25. Breithardt G, Borggrefe M: Pathophysiologic mechanisms and clinical significance of ventricular late potentials. *Eur Heart J* 7:364–385, 1986.

26. von Leitner ER, Oeff M, Loock D, Jahns B, Schröder R: Value of noninvasively detected delayed ventricular depolarizations to predict prognosis in postmyocardial infarction patient (abstr). *Circulation* 68(suppl):III-83, 1983.

27. Denniss AR, Richards DA, Cody DV, et al: Prognostic significance of ventricular tachycardia and fibrillation induced at programmed stimulation and delayed potentials detected on the signal-averaged electrocardiograms of survivors of acute myocardial infarction. *Circulation* 74:731–745, 1986.

28. Kuchar DL, Thorburn CW, Sammel NL: Prediction of serious arrhythmic events after myocardial infarction: signal-averaged electrocardiogram, Holter monitoring and radionuclide ventriculography. *J Am Coll Cardiol* 9:531–538, 1987.

29. Gomes JA, Winters SL, Stewart D, Horowitz S, Milner M, Barreca P: A new noninvasive index to predict sustained ventricular tachycardia and sudden death in the first year after myocardial infarction: based on signal-averaged electrocardiogram, radionuclide ejection fraction and Holter monitoring. *J Am Coll Cardiol* 10:349–357, 1987.

30. Cripps T, Bennett ED, Camm AJ, Ward DE: High gain signal averaged electrocardiogram combined with 24 hour monitoring in patients early after myocardial infarction for bedside prediction of arrhythmic events. *Br Heart J* 60:181–187, 1988.

31. Verzoni A, Romano S, Pozzoni L, Tarricone D, Sangiorgio S, Croce L: Prognostic significance and evolution of late ventricular potentials in the first year after myocardial infarction: a prospective study. *Pacing Clin Electrophysiol* 12:41–51, 1989.

32. Gomes JA, Winters SL, Martinson M, Machac J, Stewart D, Targonski A: The prognostic significance of quantitative signal-averaged variables related to clinical variables, site of myocardial infarction, ejection fraction and ventricular premature beats: a prospective study. *J Am Coll Cardiol* 13:377–384, 1989.

33. Malik M, Kulakowski P, Odemuyiwa O, et al: Effect of thrombolytic therapy on the predictive value of signal-averaged electrocardiography after acute myocardial infarction. *Am J Cardiol* 70:21–25, 1992.

34. de Chillou C, Rodriguez LM, Doevendans P, et al: Effects on the signal-averaged electrocardiogram of opening the coronary artery by thrombolytic therapy or percutaneous transluminal coronary angioplasty during acute myocardial infarction. *Am J Cardiol* 71:805–809, 1993.

7

QT Dispersion

Ian P. Clements, MD

Definition of QT Dispersion

QT dispersion refers to the range of QT intervals observed on the standard 12-lead electrocardiogram (ECG) (Figure 1). Measurement of the QT interval is difficult, particularly when the U wave is present. The end of the T wave is defined as the return of the T wave to the T-P baseline. When U waves are present, Day et al[1] have chosen to measure the end of the Q wave as the nadir between the T and U waves. If the end of the T wave cannot be observed in a particular lead, that lead is excluded from analysis. All 12 leads on the ECG are assessed and, if possible, the QT intervals of three ECG complexes from each lead are averaged. Kautzner et al[2] studied the reproducibility of measurements of QT dispersion in healthy subjects and found that they were more variable and less reproducible than measurements of the QT interval. These authors concluded that the inferior reproducibility of QT dispersion may limit its usefulness in risk stratification studies. Also, QT dispersion may be greater in men than in women.[3]

Clinical Significance

The rationale for ascribing clinical significance to QT dispersion derives from the known clinical significance of the QT interval. It is well recognized that prolongation of the QT interval is associated with serious arrhythmias, such as torsades de pointes and ventricular tachycardia. It is believed that these conditions are associated with increased disper-

From: Clements, IP (ed). *The Electrocardiogram in Acute Myocardial Infarction.* Armonk, NY: Futura Publishing Company, Inc. © Mayo Foundation 1998.

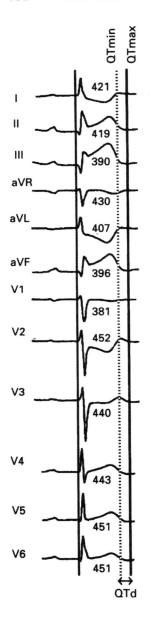

Figure 1. ECG of a patient with acute inferior infarction, showing dispersion of the QT intervals. QT dispersion (QTd) = QT_{max} (V2)—QT_{min} (V1). (Reproduced with permission from Reference 16.)

sion of ventricular recovery time. Cowan et al[4] studied differences in regional repolarization from the epicardium and found that these epicardial differences were related to the surface ECG. Prolongation of the QT interval can occur in the presence of the congenital prolongation of the QT interval, after myocardial infarction, and with certain antiarrhythmic drugs.

Analysis of QT dispersion in patients with congenitally long QT syndromes demonstrated that the QT interval is not only prolonged in these patients, but that the variation in this interval in the ECG leads is marked.[1] The rate-corrected QT interval in a group of 10 patients with predominantly congenital long QT syndrome and ventricular arrhythmia was 645 ± 32 milliseconds and the rate-corrected QT dispersion was 178 ± 18 milliseconds. This compares with the normal value of 32 ± 8 milliseconds for QT dispersion.[5]

The significance of prolonged QT dispersion was also demonstrated in a group of patients with documented sustained ventricular fibrillation or ventricular tachycardia.[5] Independently of whether the patient had chronic ischemic heart disease, cardiomyopathy, or ventricular tachycardia in a normal heart, QT dispersion was greater in patients with ventricular tachyarrhythmia than in a similar group of patients who had no history of ventricular tachyarrhythmia.

Acute Myocardial Infarction

Cowan et al[6] have demonstrated that QT dispersion is more marked in patients with acute infarction, both anterior (70 ± 30 milliseconds) and inferior (73 ± 32 milliseconds), than in control subjects (48 ± 18 milliseconds) (Figure 2). A recent study documented that the admission ECG in patients with acute myocardial infarction showed greater QT dispersion than in patients without cardiac disease (56 ± 24 milliseconds vs 30 ± 10 milliseconds).[7] Furthermore, the 11 patients in whom ventricular fibrillation developed had a longer mean QT dispersion than those without fibrillation (88 ± 30 milliseconds vs 55 ± 21 milliseconds) (Figure 3). This has been confirmed in other studies.[8,9]

Schwartz and Wolf,[10] using serial ECGs, prospectively showed that patients with acute myocardial infarction in whom ventricular fibrillation develops have prolonged QT dispersion even before ventricular fibrillation develops, in comparison with patients with infarction who remain rhythmically stable (Figure 4).

Few reported studies have attempted to show that QT dispersion has prognostic significance in acute myocardial infarction. Over a 2-year period, Zareba et al,[11] in an analysis of patients enrolled in the Multicenter Study of Myocardial Ischemia, identified 17 patients with arrhythmic cardiac death (Figure 5). These patients were matched with a group of 51 survivors. A measure of dispersion of repolarization, JT

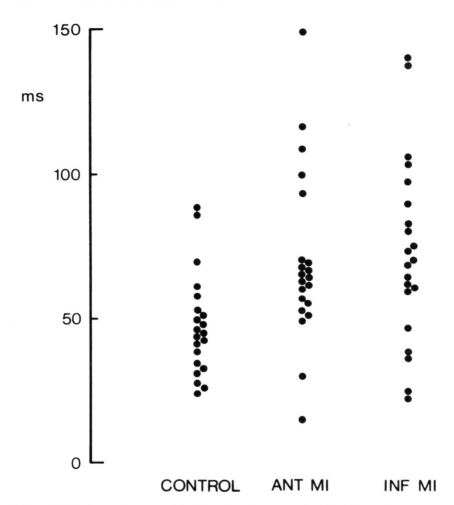

Figure 2. QT dispersion (y-axis) in 63 patients: 21 controls, 21 with anterior myocardial infarction (ANT MI), and 21 with inferior myocardial infarction (INF MI). (Reproduced with permission from Reference 6.)

dispersion, rather than QT dispersion was associated with arrhythmic cardiac death. Also, the greater the JT dispersion, the greater the risk of arrhythmic cardiac death. This variable also was an independent predictor of arrhythmic cardiac death and formed the best predictive model when combined with QRS duration (χ^2, *25.1*; $P < 0.0001$). Among the 17 deaths, 14 had JT dispersion of 80 milliseconds or more or a QRS duration of 95 milliseconds or more.

Barr et al[12] followed 44 patients with congestive heart failure due to chronic coronary artery disease. Seven patients died suddenly and 12 died of progressive congestive heart failure. QT dispersion was greater in the patients who died suddenly (99 milliseconds; 95% CI, 79 to 118 milliseconds) than in those who died of congestive heart failure (67 milliseconds; 95% CI, 52 to 82 milliseconds) or who survived (53 milliseconds; 95% CI, 42 to 64 milliseconds). Glancy et al[13] found that QT dispersion recorded 2 to 4 days after the onset of infarction was not different between survivors and nonsurvivors. These patients were followed for 4 years. However, on ECGs recorded at least 28 days after

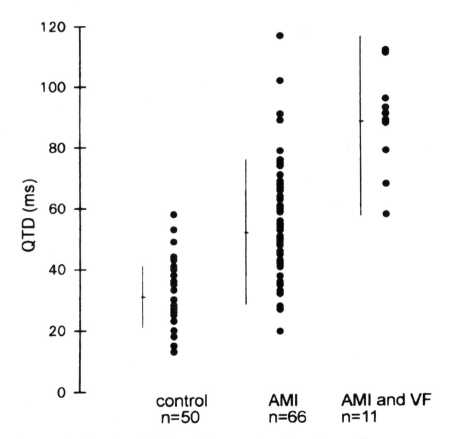

Figure 3. QT dispersion (QTD) (y-axis) in controls and in patients with acute myocardial infarction (AMI) or acute myocardial infarction and ventricular fibrillation (AMI and VF). Mean values were significantly different between the groups ($P < 0.01$). (Reproduced with permission from Reference 7.)

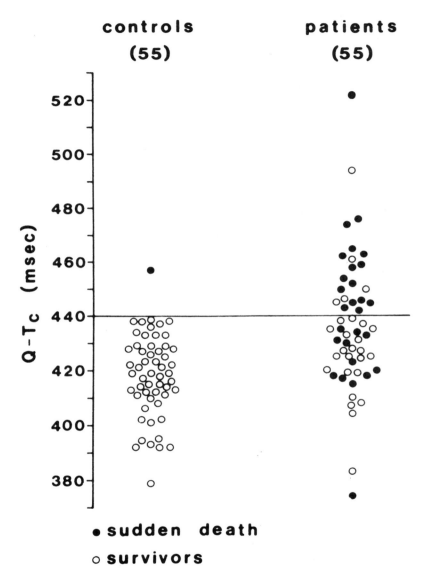

Figure 4. Distribution of corrected QT interval (Q-T$_c$) values among patients and controls. (Reproduced with permission from Reference 10.)

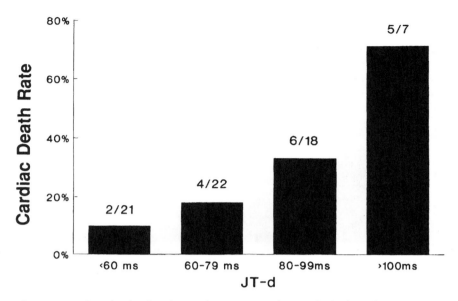

Figure 5. Cardiac death related to JT dispersion (JT-d). **Fractions above bars** represent the number of arrhythmic cardiac deaths per number of patients in each JT-d group. (Reproduced with permission from Reference 11.)

infarction, survivors had shortened QT dispersion in comparison with nonsurvivors (76.5 ± 28.8 milliseconds vs 98.9 ± 43.1 milliseconds).

Both of these latter studies suggested that variability in the dispersion of repolarization could be used for prognostic purposes in coronary artery disease and congestive heart failure.

Therapeutic Effects on QT Dispersion

Therapeutic measures do influence QT dispersion. Day et al[14] studied the effects of the class III antiarrhythmic agent, sotalol, on QT dispersion in 67 patients after myocardial infarction in comparison with placebo. Not unexpectedly, sotalol prolonged the QT interval in comparison with placebo, but QT dispersion was decreased by sotalol, as compared with placebo. It is unproved that a decrease in QT dispersion after myocardial infarction is associated with enhanced prognosis.

QT dispersion was also analyzed in relation to thrombolysis.[15] Successful thrombolysis, considered as Thrombolysis in Myocardial Infarction (TIMI) grade 3 flow, after treatment with streptokinase was associated with less QT and JT dispersion. QT dispersion was 96 ± 31, 68 ± 25, 60 ± 22, and 52 ± 19 milliseconds ($P \leq 0.0001$), and JT disper-

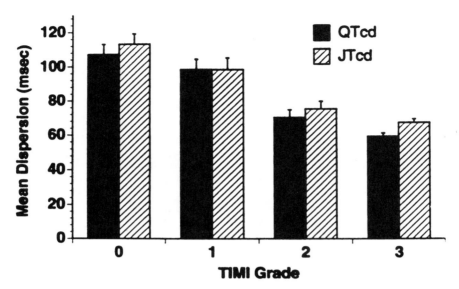

Figure 6. Dispersions of the corrected QT (QT$_{cd}$) and JT (JT$_{cd}$) intervals among patients in the four Thromboloysis in Myocardial Infarction (TIMI) perfusion groups. These differences were significant (P = 0.0001 for both QT$_{cd}$ and JT$_{cd}$ dispersion). (Reproduced with permission from Reference 15.)

sion was 97 ± 32, 88 ± 31, 63 ± 23, and 58 ± 21 milliseconds (P = 0.0001), among TIMI perfusion grades 0, 1, 2, and 3, respectively (Figure 6). These authors suggested that a reduction in QT dispersion with successful reperfusion following myocardial infarction and the potential reduction in arrhythmic death is one of the mechanisms for benefit following thrombolytic therapy.

Conclusion

Clearly, more study is required to substantiate the value of QT dispersion as a predictor of cardiac death. The day-to-day variability in the measurement of QT dispersion may be a major difficulty with its use as a predictive index. Better measurement techniques might circumvent this difficulty. However, more information about the sensitivity, specificity, and predictive accuracy for cardiac death of QT dispersion is required. Also, it needs to be established whether a reduction in QT dispersion with therapy leads to protection against arrhythmic cardiac death.[16]

References

1. Day CP, McComb JM, Campbell RW: QT dispersion: an indication of arrhythmia risk in patients with long QT intervals. *Br Heart J* 63:342–344, 1990.
2. Kautzner J, Yi G, Camm AJ, Malik M: Short- and long-term reproducibility of QT, QTc, and QT dispersion measurement in healthy subjects. *Pacing Clin Electrophysiol* 17:928–937, 1994.
3. Fei L, Statters DJ, Camm AJ: QT-interval dispersion on 12-lead electrocardiogram in normal subjects: its reproducibility and relation to the T wave. *Am Heart J* 127:1654–1655, 1994.
4. Cowan JC, Hilton CJ, Griffiths CJ, et al: Sequence of epicardial repolarisation and configuration of the T wave. *Br Heart J* 60:424–433, 1988.
5. Pye M, Quinn AC, Cobbe SM: QT interval dispersion: a non-invasive marker of susceptibility to arrhythmias in patients with sustained ventricular arrhythmias? *Br Heart J* 71:511–514, 1994.
6. Cowan JC, Yusoff K, Moore M, et al: Importance of lead selection in QT interval measurement. *Am J Cardiol* 61:83–87, 1988.
7. van de Loo A, Arendts W, Hohnloser SH: Variability of QT dispersion measurements in the surface electrocardiogram in patients with acute myocardial infarction and in normal subjects. *Am J Cardiol* 74:1113–1118, 1994.
8. Bashir Y, Farrell TG, Camm AJ: Increased QT dispersion in survivors of acute myocardial infarction who subsequently develop ventricular arrhythmias or sudden death (abstr). *Pacing Clin Electrophysiol* 13:561, 1990.
9. Higham PD, Furniss SS, Campbell RWF: Increased QT dispersion in patients with ventricular fibrillation following myocardial infarction (abstr). *Circulation* 84(suppl 2):61, 1991.
10. Schwartz PJ, Wolf S: QT interval prolongation as predictor of sudden death in patients with myocardial infarction. *Circulation* 57:1074–1077, 1978.
11. Zareba W, Moss AJ, le Cessie S: Dispersion of ventricular repolarization and arrhythmic cardiac death in coronary artery disease. *Am J Cardiol* 74:550–553, 1994.
12. Barr CS, Nass A, Freeman M, Lang CC, Struthers AD: QT dispersion and sudden unexpected death in chronic heart failure. *Lancet* 343:327–329, 1994.
13. Glancy JM, Garratt CJ, Woods KL, de Bono DP: QT dispersion and mortality after myocardial infarction. *Lancet* 345:945–948, 1995.
14. Day CP, McComb JM, Matthews J, Campbell RW: Reduction in QT dispersion by sotalol following myocardial infarction. *Eur Heart J* 12:423–427, 1991.
15. Moreno FL, Villanueva T, Karagounis LA, Anderson JL: Reduction in QT interval dispersion by successful thrombolytic therapy in acute myocardial infarction. *Circulation* 90:94–100, 1994.
16. Higham PD, Campbell RW: QT dispersion. *Br Heart J* 71:508–510, 1994.

8

The High-Frequency Electrocardiogram

Ian P. Clements, MD

Because the voltage changes in the usual electrocardiogram (ECG) occur at low frequencies, the high-frequency component (>100 Hz) is eliminated by filtering. However, several investigators have analyzed the high-frequency components of the ECG (100 to 1,000 Hz).[1] It has been suggested that certain features of these high-frequency ECGs can be used for the diagnosis of myocardial infarction.[1,2]

To generate these high-frequency ECGs, a number of signal-processing steps that involve high-gain amplification and signal filtering and averaging take place. The result of this process is the generation of a signal-averaged high-frequency QRS complex (Figure 1). A further signal-processing step is performed and an envelope is placed around the resulting high-frequency signal. In normal subjects, this envelope is smooth and no reduced amplitude zone is noted within the envelope.

High-frequency ECGs have been analyzed in experimental and clinical settings in acute myocardial infarction. In dogs, occlusion of the left anterior descending coronary artery produced a zone of reduced amplitude in the high-frequency signal within 30 to 45 seconds after the occlusion; this zone disappeared with reperfusion (Figure 2).[3] The changes were thought to occur within a few beats after occlusion.

The high-frequency ECG has been studied before, during, and after balloon inflation in patients. Abboud et al[4] noted several features on these ECGs (Figure 3). First, there was a decline in cross correlation between the high-frequency ECGs in the control patients and those who had balloon inflation; this commenced within a few beats after inflation

From: Clements, IP (ed). *The Electrocardiogram in Acute Myocardial Infarction.* Armonk, NY: Futura Publishing Company, Inc. © Mayo Foundation 1998.

and much earlier than the changes seen in the ST segment and T wave. Second, the root-mean-square of the high-frequency QRS signal decreased with balloon inflation. Third, a zone of reduced amplitude was seen in the high-frequency QRS signal. These three changes promptly reverted to baseline after balloon deflation (Figure 4). It should be noted that this was not always the typical pattern with balloon inflation. A zone of reduced amplitude was present in 9 of 11 patients before balloon inflation. A zone of reduced amplitude developed in only two patients with balloon inflation. However, balloon inflation was associated with a reduction in the root-mean-square voltage of the high-frequency signal in all the patients.

Abboud et al[5] also analyzed the high-frequency QRS signal during reperfusion with thrombolytic agents in nine patients with a first myocardial infarction. The authors observed that successful thrombolysis was associated with an increase in the root-mean-square of the high-frequency signal, whereas persistent occlusion was associated with a further decrease (Figures 5A and 5B). Abboud et al[5] suggested that the changes in the high-frequency ECG may be used to detect successful reperfusion in acute myocardial infarction.

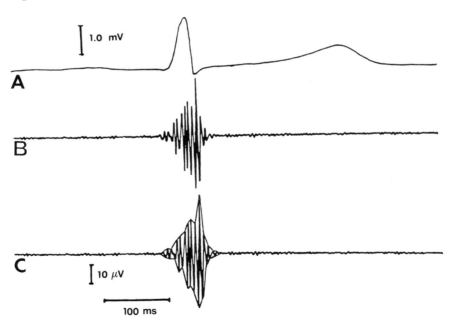

Figure 1. Signal-averaged nonfiltered ECG of surface lead V₅ (**A**), the signal-averaged high-frequency (150–250 Hz) QRS complex (**B**), and the computer-generated delineation of the envelope of the high-frequency QRS complex (**C**) from a normal subject. (Reproduced with permission from Reference 4.)

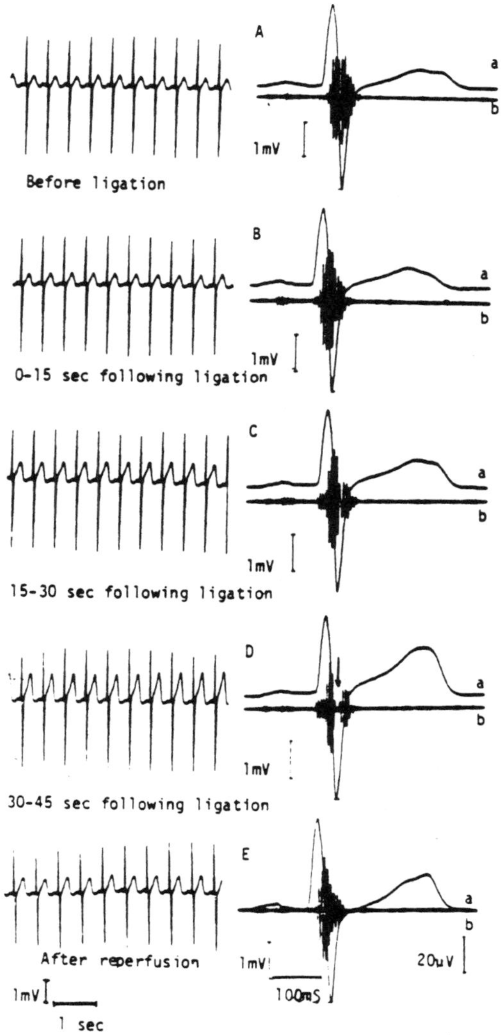

Figure 2. A-E. Sequential tracings of lead Z in a dog during different stages of coronary artery ligation. The **tracings** on the **left** are the raw ECG data, and those on the **right** are the averaged nonfiltered (**a**) and filtered (**b**) high-frequency waveforms. With coronary artery occlusion, the area of high-frequency on the filtered waveforms decreased and a zone of reduced amplitude appeared (**arrow** in trace D). These changes were reversed with reperfusion. (Reproduced with permission from Reference 3.)

Summary

Analysis of the high-frequency component of the QRS complex may be useful in detecting myocardial ischemia and reperfusion. Experimental myocardial ischemia causes a reduction in the root-mean-square of the high-frequency component of the ECG and occasional separation of the component into two regions. Reperfusion reverses these changes.

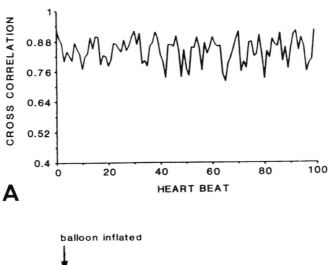

A

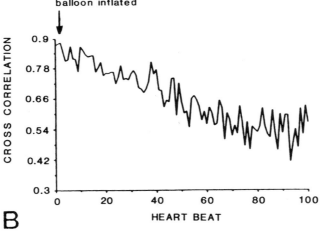

B

Figure 3. Beat-to-beat variation in the high-frequency (150 to 250 Hz) QRS complexes obtained before and during coronary artery occlusion in a dog. The vertical axis represents the normalized cross-correlation coefficient between the high-frequency QRS complex from a reference template and that of subsequent waveforms. **A.** No change in correlation was noted before occlusion but **B.**, correlation decreased within several beats after occlusion. (Reproduced with permission from Abboud S: Subtle alterations in the high-frequency QRS potentials during myocardial ischemia in dogs. *Comput Biomed Res* 20:384–395, 1987.)

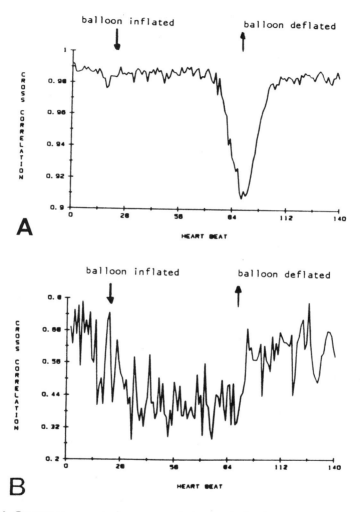

Figure 4. Computer-generated cross-correlation analysis of ST-segment and T-wave morphology of the standard surface ECG (**A**) and the nonaveraged high-frequency QRS complex in lead V_5 (**B**) during percutaneous transluminal coronary angioplasty (PTCA). Cross correlation decreased earlier after PTCA for the high-frequency QRS components (**B**) compared with ST-segment and T-wave morphology. For both curves, there was a prompt return to baseline after balloon deflation. (Reproduced with permission from Reference 4.)

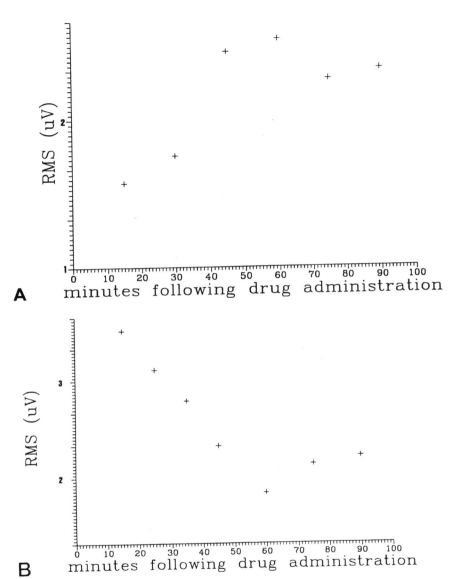

Figure 5. Root mean square (RMS) voltage of the high-frequency QRS complexes recorded from a patient with a myocardial infarction who had successful reperfusion (**A**) and a patient without reperfusion (**B**). Reperfusion was associated with an increase in RMS voltage of the high-frequency component, whereas failure to reperfuse was associated with a decline in RMS voltage of this component. (**A** reproduced with permission from Reference 1; **B** reproduced with permission from Reference 5.)

These features are produced in patients during balloon occlusion of the coronary artery before angioplasty. The most constant feature of coronary artery occlusion in the high-frequency ECG is the reduction in root-mean-square of the high-frequency component.

In patients with acute infarction, reperfusion has been observed to increase the root-mean-square of the high-frequency QRS component.

Further study of the high-frequency component of the QRS complex is necessary to determine whether these observations could be of value in detecting infarct-related artery reperfusion in the clinical setting.

References

1. Abboud S: High-frequency electrocardiogram analysis of the entire QRS in the diagnosis and assessment of coronary artery disease. *Prog Cardiovasc Dis* 35: 311–328, 1993.
2. Goldberger AL, Bhargava V, Froelicher V, Covell J: Effect of myocardial infarction on high-frequency QRS potentials. *Circulation* 64:34–42, 1981.
3. Abboud S, Smith JM, Shargorodsky B, Laniado S, Sadeh D, Cohen RJ: High frequency electrocardiography of three orthogonal leads in dogs during a coronary artery occlusion. *Pacing Clin Electrophysiol* 12:574–581, 1989.
4. Abboud S, Cohen RJ, Selwyn A, Ganz P, Sadeh D, Friedman PL: Detection of transient myocardial ischemia by computer analysis of standard and signal-averaged high-frequency electrocardiograms in patients undergoing percutaneous transluminal coronary angioplasty. *Circulation* 76:585–596, 1987.
5. Abboud S, Leor J, Eldar M: High-frequency ECG during reperfusion therapy of acute myocardial infarction. IEEE Computer Society, *Computers in Cardiology* 351–352, 1990.

9

Variance Electrocardiography

Ian P. Clements, MD

The QRS portion of the electrocardiogram (ECG) has been analyzed for beat-to-beat variation in electrical potential.[1-5] It is argued that this variation occurs when myocardial scarring or abnormality is present and causes beat-to-beat variation in the pathway of myocardial depolarization. Thus, detection of this beat-to-beat variation will indicate abnormal myocardium. This hypothesis has been applied in patients with myocardial infarction and coronary artery disease.[2-5]

One technique involves recording the ECG signals from 22 skin and thoracic electrodes, 10 of which are the same as those of the standard 12-lead ECG.[3-5] Low-pass filtering (0.05 Hz to 1,500 Hz), voltage amplification, and digitization are performed, and 220 ECG complexes are acquired. Ectopic activity and noise are excluded. Each beat from each ECG lead is compared with a template constructed from the recorded beats, and the variation from the template is calculated. The calculated variation of the ECG complexes in each lead is summated, and a variance index is generated. The variance index provides an estimate of the variation of the QRS configuration. The greater the value of the variance index, the less likely a patient is to have a normal myocardium.

The variance index has been determined in patients with a low risk of coronary artery disease,[1] with coronary artery disease,[2] or with acute myocardial infarction.[3] For patients with a low risk of coronary artery disease, the variance index was 57.4 $\pm$ 18.5 (range, 6 to 116). Fifteen of these patients had a variance index greater than 75 (range, 75 to 116). In 8 of these 15 patients, a tomographic thallium image was abnormal. When 181 patients with angiographically documented coronary artery

From: Clements, IP (ed). *The Electrocardiogram in Acute Myocardial Infarction.* Armonk, NY: Futura Publishing Company, Inc. © Mayo Foundation 1998.

disease were studied, the variance index was 90.7 ± 19.7 (range, 50 to 149), which was significantly greater than that in low-risk patients.[2]

In 41 patients admitted and subsequently documented by cardiac enzyme studies to have an acute myocardial infarction, a variance score of ≥ 85, obtained within a mean of 6 to 7 hours after the onset of infarction, had a sensitivity of 83% for detecting myocardial infarction, whereas the standard 12-lead ECG had a sensitivity of only 51%.[3] In the same study, the variance score of 74 patients with chest pain who subsequently were shown by cardiac enzyme studies not to have a myocardial infarction had a specificity of 76%, which was lower than that of the 12-lead ECG (99%).

These findings indicate that a variance score of ≥ 85 has a positive predictive value of 65% and a negative predictive value of 89% for myocardial infarction, in comparison with values of 96% and 79%, respectively, for the standard 12-lead ECG.

The major difficulty in using the variance ECG as a discriminator of the presence or absence of myocardial infarction is that the variance ECG is abnormal in patients with coronary artery disease.[2-5] This finding decreases the specificity of the variance score in detecting the absence of myocardial infarction. The variance ECG, however, appears to be as accurate as myocardial scintigraphy in detecting coronary artery disease and is superior to the stress ECG.[4,5]

Ben-Haim and coworkers,[6] with a different technique, also studied the variation in beat-to-beat morphology in a group of patients with healed myocardial infarction. Variance determinations were made at the onset and offset of the QRS complex. A significant difference in variance was found at QRS onset (60- to 120-Hz-filtered ECG) and offset (4- to 40-Hz-filtered ECG) when normal volunteers were compared with patients with healed myocardial infarctions (Figure 1).

The beat-to-beat variation in the ECG was also analyzed by Prasad and coworkers,[7,8] who used the phase-invariant signature algorithm (PISA) to analyze the ECG signal in the phase domain. In normal subjects, myocardial depolarization generally should be uniform. Thus, in the phase domain in normal subjects, the ECG does not vary and is said to be "phase-invariant." However, in the presence of myocardial abnormality, such as in ischemic heart disease or hypertension, in which the depolarization wave can randomly take one of many different pathways, the ECG varies in the phase domain (Figure 2). This variation can be quantified as the PISA index.

---→

Figure 1. A. Beat-to-beat relative variance of high-frequency (60- to 120-Hz)-filtered ECG signal compared between normal subjects and patients with myocardial ischemia. * $P < 0.005$. **B.** Beat-to-beat relative variance of low-frequency (4- to 40-Hz)-filtered ECG signal compared between normal subjects and patients with myocardial ischemia. * $P < 0.02$. (Reproduced with permission from Reference 6.)

QRS ONSET - RELATIVE VARIANCE

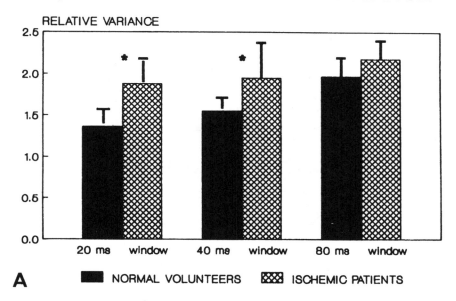

A

QRS OFFSET - RELATIVE VARIANCE

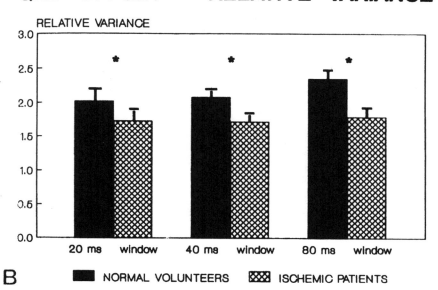

B

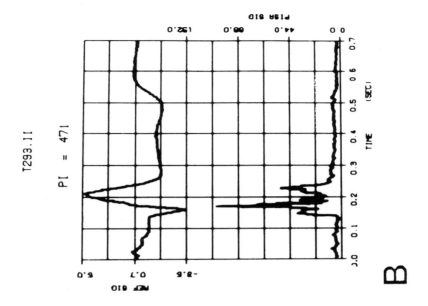

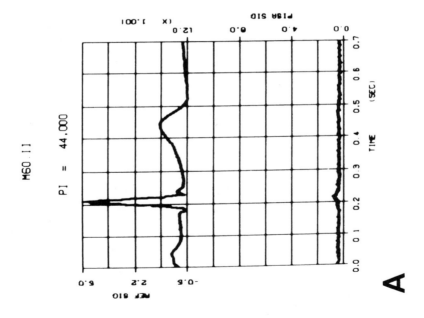

Conclusion

Statistical analysis of the beat-to-beat variation in the QRS of the ECG indicates that increased variation occurs in the presence of myocardial lesions, including coronary artery disease, myocardial infarction, and hypertension. The overlap in variance between various myocardial disorders may limit the usefulness of ECG variance analysis for the detection of acute myocardial infarction.

References

1. Gobel FL, Tschida VH: Screening yield of electrocardiogram chaos analysis in low-risk asymptomatic individuals (abstr). *Circulation* 82(suppl 3):III-619, 1990.
2. Tschida VH, Gobel FL: Accuracy of electrocardiogram chaos analysis for the diagnosis of coronary artery disease (abstr). *Circulation* 82(suppl 3):III-236, 1990.
3. Justis DL, Hession WT: Accuracy of 22-lead ECG analysis for diagnosis of acute myocardial infarction and coronary artery disease in the emergency department: a comparison with 12-lead ECG. *Ann Emerg Med* 21:1–9, 1992.
4. Nowak J, Hagerman I, Ylen M, Nyquist O, Sylven C: Electrocardiogram signal variance analysis in the diagnosis of coronary artery disease—a comparison with exercise stress test in an angiographically documented high prevalence population. *Clin Cardiol* 16:671–682, 1993.
5. Sylven C, Hagerman I, Ylen M, Nyquist O, Nowak J: Variance ECG detection of coronary artery disease—a comparison with exercise stress test and myocardial scintigraphy. *Clin Cardiol* 17:132–140, 1994.
6. Ben-Haim SA, Becker B, Edoute Y, et al: Beat-to-beat electrocardiographic morphology variation in healed myocardial infarction. *Am J Cardiol* 68:725–728, 1991.
7. Prasad K, Gupta MM: Phase-invariant signature algorithm: a noninvasive technique for early detection and quantification of ouabain-induced cardiac disorders. *Angiology* 30:721–732, 1979.
8. Prasad K, Gupta MM, Nikiforuk PN, et al: PISA—a new noninvasive method for early detection and quantification of ischemia in hypertensive patients. *Angiology* 36:75–87, 1985.

←―――――――――――――――――――――――――――――――――――――――

Figure 2. A typical tracing from a healthy subject (**A**) and a person with ischemic heart disease (**B**). In each panel, the **top tracing** is the reference signal (REF SIG), which is an ensemble average of wide-band electrocardiac signals of 60 cardiac cycles. The **bottom tracing** is its corresponding PISA signature (PISA SIG). PI = PISA index. Note that the healthy person has a straight-line PISA signature and small PISA index of 44. The person with ischemic heart disease has a nonstraight-line PISA signature and a high PISA index of 471. (Reproduced with permission from Reference 8.)

Limitations of Standard 12-Lead Electrocardiogram in Detecting Acute Myocardial Infarction

Timothy F. Christian, MD

Introduction

Advances in therapy have had an important effect on the outcome of acute myocardial infarction. Intravenous thrombolytic therapy has decreased 30-day mortality to 4% to 8% for patients who receive treatment within 6 hours after the onset of symptoms.[1-4] The decrease in mortality, as compared with that of patients receiving placebo, has ranged from 16% to 50%, using various agents and dosages.[1-4] Direct coronary angioplasty also has been shown to be highly effective for the treatment of acute myocardial infarction.[5,6] The mortality for small randomized trials of this therapy has been low, 2.0% to 2.6%. However, all these trials that showed a clear benefit for intervention were conducted in highly selected populations. Most notably, all the patients who were included presented with symptoms in a timely manner and all had diagnostic ST-segment elevation consistent with acute injury.

However, in the world of clinical practice, matters are not so simple. Patients often have symptoms that wax and wane, making the timing of the occlusion imprecise. Also, the occlusion process is dynamic, with cyclical occlusion and recanalization.[7] Yet, the criteria of diagnostic ST-segment elevation is relied on as a key factor in determining who receives reperfusion therapy and who does not. This chapter considers

From: Clements, IP (ed). *The Electrocardiogram in Acute Myocardial Infarction.* Armonk, NY: Futura Publishing Company, Inc. © Mayo Foundation 1998.

what is known about the performance of this simple measurement as an indicator of acute myocardial infarction.

Genesis of ST-Segment Injury Current

The degree of ST-segment elevation is the product of two factors: the extent of ischemia (spatial influences) and the severity of ischemia (non-spatial influences).[8] In ischemia, the resting transmembrane potential of ischemic cells is less negative than that of nonischemic cells. After depolarization, the situation is reversed. During repolarization, the ischemic zone becomes more negative than normal myocardium, probably because of incomplete depolarization. The additive impact of these factors (resting TQ depression and systolic ST-segment elevation) produces the magnitude of ST-segment elevation.[8] In a simplistic manner, then, the spatial extent of ischemia could be measured by the number of leads with ST deflection and the severity of ischemia could be measured by the amount of deflection. A number of factors mitigate this simple relationship.

The conductance within the thorax varies depending on the organs between the myocardium and the recording electrode, and this influences the magnitude of the deflections. Also, the thorax is not circular; therefore, the distance from the myocardium to an electrode varies with location. Most importantly, the territories within the myocardium are not equally represented by the standard 12-lead electrocardiogram (ECG). ST-segment elevation is produced by a gradient of current between ischemic (negative) and normal (positive) myocardium during repolarization, causing the overlying electrode to record a "positive" deflection. However, the posterolateral wall of the left ventricle has no overlying electrode. Consequently, ST-segment elevation usually does not occur with this type of infarction and is said to be "electrically silent."

Myocardial Infarction in the Absence of ST-Segment Elevation

This phenomenon of an "electrically silent" zone has been demonstrated repeatedly in clinical trials of acute myocardial infarction. There is nothing intrinsically different about the left circumflex artery that would predispose it to a lower propensity for plaque rupture and thrombus formation. However, it is consistently under-represented in clinical trials of myocardial infarction.[4,5] The angiographic substudy of the Global Utilization of Streptokinase and Tissue Plasminogen Activator for Occluded Coronary Arteries (GUSTO) trial found that the left circumflex artery was identified as the culprit vessel in only 12% of the patients enrolled,[9] which is in contrast to 39% and 44% for left anterior descending and right coronary artery occlusion, respectively. This trial required patients to have at least 2 mV of ST-segment elevation in two limb leads or 2 mV in two contiguous precordial leads. Other clinical trials have shown a similar under-representation of left circumflex artery occlusion.[10–12]

The majority of patients who present with acute myocardial infarction do not have diagnostic ST-segment elevation on the acute 12-lead ECG. In the Multicenter Chest Pain Study that included more than 1,000 patients with myocardial infarction, only 45% had diagnostic ST-segment elevation (Figure 1).[13] The majority of patients had a combination of ST-segment depression, nonspecific changes, or marked conduction disturbance that prevented adequate analysis of the presenting ECG. In 7% of the patients, the ECG was completely normal despite the occurrence of acute myocardial infarction.

These findings were similar to those reported from the William

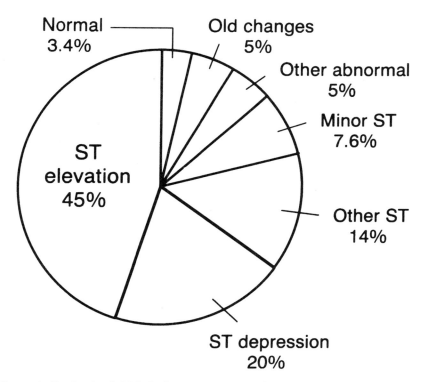

Figure 1. Twelve-lead ECG findings in patients who presented to an emergency department with chest pain and in whom myocardial infarction was subsequently documented. (Data reproduced from Reference 13.)

Beaumont Hospital.[14] Nearly one half of the patients presenting with chest pain in whom myocardial infarction was subsequently documented did not have the ST-segment elevation needed to meet the eligibility requirements for thrombolytic therapy. These findings were not without consequence. The mortality for those who had ECGs that met the eligibility requirements for thrombolysis and who subsequently received such treatment was 4%, but for those with ineligible ECGs, the rate was more than threefold higher, 14% (Figure 2).

ECG Criteria for Diagnosis of Myocardial Infarction

The accuracy of the 12-lead ECG in diagnosing acute myocardial infarction is a function of the criteria used. The Multicenter Investigation of the Limitation of Infarct Size (MILIS) trial analyzed the ECGs of 3,697 patients presenting with more than 30 minutes of chest pain.[15] Table 1 demonstrates the performance of the ECG in correctly ruling in or out the presence of acute myocardial infarction. Dependence on significant ST-segment elevation alone resulted in a high specificity of 91% (correct identification of those without acute myocardial infarction), but a low sensitivity of 46% (correct identification of those with acute myocardial infarction). The performance in unselected populations was even lower.[16] The performance of the ECG incrementally improves as the criteria are broadened, but because of the potential complications of thrombolytic therapy in those without active coronary thrombosis, most clinical trials have been unwilling to accept these wider criteria.

It is clear from several studies that the usual criteria for giving thrombolytic therapy are inadvertently biased against patients presenting with isolated left circumflex artery occlusion. Huey et al[12] compared a cohort of patients who had myocardial infarction due to left circumflex artery occlusion with those who had isolated occlusion of the right coronary or left anterior descending artery. Only 48% of patients with left circumflex artery occlusion had ST-segment elevation on the acute ECG, a prevalence of ST-segment elevation that was significantly less than the prevalence of ST-segment elevations associated with infarction in the other two vascular territories. Abnormal R waves were present in only 50% of patients, and anterior ST-segment depression was present in 45%. Nondiagnostic ECGs (no ST-segment elevation or depression) were present in 38% of patients with left circumflex occlusion.[12]

The diminished sensitivity of ST-segment elevation for left circumflex artery occlusion appears to be due primarily to the limitations of the 12-lead surface ECG. Berry et al[17] performed intracoronary ECG during elective coronary angioplasty in patients and found that the degree of ST-segment elevation was similar among the three major vessels. However, there was a marked disparity when the surface ECG was ana-

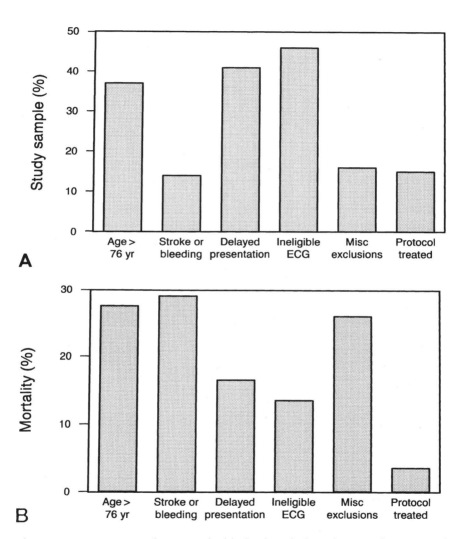

Figure 2. A. Percentages of patients eligible for thrombolytic therapy who presented with acute myocardial infarction (protocol-treated) and the prevalence of various reasons for withholding such therapy. **B.** Mortality rate for each category of patients. (Reproduced with permission from Reference 14.)

Table 1
Sensitivity and Specificity of ECG Criteria in Diagnosing
Acute Myocardial Infarction

Criteria	Sensitivity, %	Specificity, %
ST-segment elevation	46	91
ST-segment elevation or depression	75	77
ST-segment elevation or depression, Q waves, or left bundle branch block	81	69

lyzed. Only 32% of patients with left circumflex artery dilatation demonstrated ST-segment elevation, as compared with 84% and 92% for patients with dilatation of the left anterior descending and right coronary arteries, respectively. Other reports have confirmed the lack of association between left circumflex artery occlusion and ST-segment elevation on the 12-lead ECG.[18,19] However, O'Keefe et al[20] have shown that reperfusion therapy of left circumflex artery occlusion without ST-segment elevation produces a degree of myocardial salvage that is not different from that of right coronary or left circumflex artery occlusion in the presence of ST-segment elevation. Randomized clinical trials have begun to include ST-segment depression in the anterior precordial leads as an indication for thrombolytic therapy.[21] However, indiscriminate use of thrombolytic therapy in patients with ST-segment depression and chest pain has been shown to be of no value and potentially harmful.[1,22] Perhaps adjunctive imaging procedures performed acutely may better guide therapy in patients with ST-segment depression.[20]

Residual Blood Flow in Myocardial Infarction

Although involvement of the left circumflex territory is responsible for a large proportion of the patients who present with nondiagnostic ECGs, there are other factors. It is now clear that the process of coronary artery occlusion is dynamic. Cyclical variation between occlusion and spontaneous thrombolysis has been observed with serial acute coronary angiography.[7] It is logical to presume that such variations in blood flow produce a spectrum of injury current as a function of time. Continuous ST-segment monitoring (described in detail elsewhere in this book) provides an opportunity to evaluate the prevalence with which such variation may exist.[23] Using this technology in patients with acute myocardial infarction, investigators have shown that ST segments transiently normalize in 33% to 50% of patients.[24,25] Usually, the normalization is repetitive. Because the standard 12-lead ECG provides only a snapshot in time, it clearly is possible that the ECG will be performed during a period of ST-segment normalization, thus misleading clinicians about the presence of acute coronary artery occlusion.

Another related factor is the presence of collateral flow. The magnitude of ST-segment elevation is determined partly by the severity of ischemia in acutely ischemic myocardium compared with normal myocardium.[8] Significant degrees of collateral flow extend the time of benefit for reperfusion therapy.[26,27] This is so because the oxygen supplied by such flow lessens the severity of ischemia. We have used angiographic and radionuclide techniques to show that the degree of collateral flow is related inversely to the magnitude of ST-segment elevation in patients with acute myocardial infarction (Figure 3).[28] Patients with the greatest degree of collateral flow have the least amount of ST-segment elevation. These same patients benefit the most from reperfusion therapy given in the 2 hours after the onset of symptoms. It is conceivable that significant degrees of collateral flow, just as with anterograde flow described above, may nearly normalize the ST-segment response. This is another factor that may lead clinicians away from the correct diagnosis.

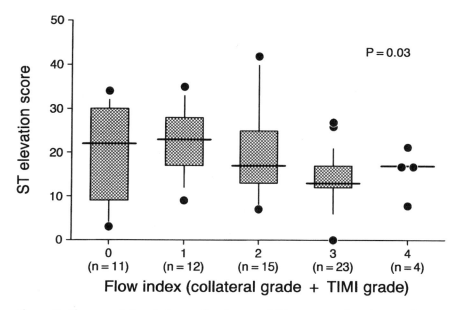

Figure 3. The association between the degree of ST-segment elevation on the 12-lead ECG and the amount of residual blood flow (anterograde or collateral or both) to the jeopardized zone in patients undergoing acute angiography prior to primary coronary angioplasty. (Reproduced with permission from Reference 28.)

Consequences of Failure to Diagnose Myocardial Infarction

It can be argued that although the diagnosis of acute myocardial infarction is missed in a number of patients because of a lack of ST-segment elevation, the consequences are small since these represent small infarctions. Experimental observation has shown that this is an incorrect assumption. We have found by using technetium Tc 99m sestamibi acute perfusion imaging that the amount of jeopardized myocardium in patients presenting with normal or nondiagnostic ECGs in whom myocardial infarction is subsequently documented is not small (Figure 4).[29] For this group of patients, the amount of myocardium at risk ranged between 20% and 51% of the left ventricle. Consistent with the discussion above, many of these patients had occlusion of the left circumflex artery, although other vascular territories were involved in some patients. The average amount of left ventricle that was involved was 21%, which is equivalent to the value obtained for patients with inferior myocardial infarction with ST-segment elevation.[29] Several patients in this study had left bundle branch block on the presenting ECG and significant amounts of myocardium at risk. Such patients present a challenge.

Patients presenting with a new or old bundle branch block during acute myocardial infarction have an exceptionally high mortality rate.

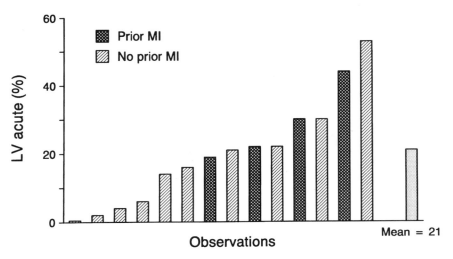

Figure 4. The extent of left ventricular (LV) myocardium at risk as measured by acute technetium Tc 99m sestamibi imaging (LV acute) in a series of patients with myocardial infarction in the absence of ST-segment elevation. A significant proportion of patients had left circumflex artery occlusion. (Reproduced from data from Reference 29.)

The ISIS-2 trial demonstrated that the 30-day mortality for such patients receiving conventional treatment was more than 25%. However, thrombolytic therapy results in a marked reduction in mortality, to 14%, in such patients.[1] Consequently, the timely diagnosis of acute infarction is of great importance in these patients. Some evidence suggests that continuous ST-segment monitoring may aid in the diagnosis of infarction, despite the marked distortion of the ST-segment from this conduction abnormality. Additionally, multiple criteria regarding the magnitude of ST-segment deviation have been reported.[30] However, in the absence of an old ECG, it probably is best to promptly administer thrombolytic therapy to these patients. If relative contraindications exist, perfusion imaging with technetium Tc 99m sestamibi or serum markers (or both) can aid in the decision process.

Sex Differences

Recently, sex-related differences in the ECG in acute myocardial infarction have been of concern. Investigators have pointed out that thrombolytic therapy after acute myocardial infarction is used less frequently in women despite the presence of similar indications. This suggests a bias that is unfavorable to women in the decision to use thrombolysis for acute myocardial infarction. The recently completed Myocardial Infarction Triage and Intervention (MITI) trial reported that 26% of eligible men received thrombolytic therapy in comparison with 14% of eligible women.[31] Some investigators point to the ECG as a potential explanation for such possible bias. Dellborg et al[32] reported from the Thrombolysis Early in Acute Heart Attack Trial (TEAHAT) study that the magnitude of ST-segment elevation as determined from dynamic ECG monitoring was significantly higher in men than in women with acute infarction. However, Raitt et al[33] could not confirm these findings on analyzing the MITI trial registry. They found no difference in the percentage of patients with diagnostic ST-segment elevation (46% of eligible men versus 43% of eligible women). There was a trend for higher maximal ST-segment elevation in men in the subset of patients with anterior infarction, but virtually no difference in inferior infarction. The thoracic wall does differ between men and women, and this may have the most impact on the anterior precordial leads. However, it does not appear that the 12-lead ECG alone is responsible for the disparate use of thrombolytic therapy according to sex.

Conclusion

It is evident that the ECG, although inexpensive and readily available, is not all we wish it to be in its performance to triage patients with chest pain syndromes. The inclusion of ST-segment depression in the anterior precordial leads to increase the diagnostic capability for patients with left circumflex artery occlusion and the prompt use of reperfusion therapy in patients with new left bundle branch block may enhance that performance. Still, this approach will fail to diagnose myocardial infarction in many patients presenting with chest pain. Given the high mortality in these patients, adjunctive measures such as rapid serum markers and cardiac imaging procedures are required to provide optimal care, although the 12-lead ECG will always have a prominent role in these situations.

References

1. ISIS-2 (Second International Study of Infarct Survival) Collaborative Group: Randomised trial of intravenous streptokinase, oral aspirin, both, or neither among 17,187 cases of suspected acute myocardial infarction: ISIS-2. *Lancet* 2: 349–360, 1988.
2. Gruppo Italiano per lo Studio della Sopravvivenza nell'Infarto Miocardico: GISSI-2: A factorial randomised trial of alteplase versus streptokinase and heparin versus no heparin among 12,490 patients with acute myocardial infarction. *Lancet* 336:65–71, 1990.
3. The TIMI Study Group: Comparison of invasive and conservative strategies after treatment with intravenous tissue plasminogen activator in acute myocardial infarction. Results of the Thrombolysis in Myocardial Infarction (TIMI) phase II trial. *N Engl J Med* 320:618–627, 1989.
4. The GUSTO Investigators: An international randomized trial comparing four thrombolytic strategies for acute myocardial infarction. *N Engl J Med* 329: 673–682, 1993.
5. Grines CL, Browne KF, Marco J, et al: A comparison of immediate angioplasty with thrombolytic therapy for acute myocardial infarction. *N Engl J Med* 328: 673–679, 1993.
6. Gibbons RJ, Holmes DR, Reeder GS, Bailey KR, Hopfenspirger MR, Gersh BJ: Immediate angioplasty compared with the administration of a thrombolytic agent followed by conservative treatment for myocardial infarction. *N Engl J Med* 328: 685–691, 1993.
7. Hackett D, Davies G, Chierchia S, Maseri A: Intermittent coronary occlusion in acute myocardial infarction. Value of combined thrombolytic and vasodilator therapy. *N Engl J Med* 317:1055–1059, 1987.
8. Holland RP, Arnsdorf MF: Solid angle theory and the electrocardiogram: physiologic and quantitative interpretations. *Prog Cardiovasc Dis* 19:431–457, 1977.
9. The GUSTO Angiographic Investigators: The effects of tissue plasminogen activator, streptokinase, or both on coronary-artery patency, ventricular function, and survival after acute myocardial infarction. *N Engl J Med* 329:1615–1622, 1993.
10. Stadius ML, Maynard C, Fritz JK, et al: Coronary anatomy and left ventricular function in the first 12 hours of acute myocardial infarction: the Western Washington Randomized Intracoronary Streptokinase Trial. *Circulation* 72:292–301, 1985.
11. Chesebro JH, Knatterud G, Roberts R, et al: Thrombolysis in Myocardial Infarc-

tion (TIMI) Trial, Phase I: a comparison between intravenous tissue plasminogen activator and intravenous streptokinase. Clinical findings through hospital discharge. *Circulation* 76:142–154, 1987.

12. Huey BL, Beller GA, Kaiser DL, Gibson RS: A comprehensive analysis of myocardial infarction due to left circumflex artery occlusion: comparison with infarction due to right coronary artery and left anterior descending artery occlusion. *J Am Coll Cardiol* 12:1156–1166, 1988.

13. Rouan GW, Lee TH, Cook EF, Brand DA, Weisberg MC, Goldman L: Clinical characteristics and outcome of acute myocardial infarction in patients with initially normal or nonspecific electrocardiograms. *Am J Cardiol* 64:1087–1092, 1989.

14. Cragg DR, Friedman HZ, Bonema JD, et al: Outcome of patients with acute myocardial infarction who are ineligible for thrombolytic therapy. *Ann Intern Med* 115:173–177, 1991.

15. Rude RE, Poole WK, Muller JE, et al: Electrocardiographic and clinical criteria for recognition of acute myocardial infarction based on analysis of 3,697 patients. *Am J Cardiol* 52:936–942, 1983.

16. Zarling EJ, Sexton H, Milnor P Jr: Failure to diagnose acute myocardial infarction. The clinicopathologic experience at a large community hospital. *JAMA* 250: 1177–1181, 1983.

17. Berry C, Zalewski A, Kovach R, Savage M, Goldberg S: Surface electrocardiogram in the detection of transmural myocardial ischemia during coronary artery occlusion. *Am J Cardiol* 63:21–26, 1989.

18. Boden WE, Kleiger RE, Gibson RS, et al: Electrocardiographic evolution of posterior acute myocardial infarction: importance of early precordial ST-segment depression. *Am J Cardiol* 59:782–787, 1987.

19. Sclarovsky S, Topas O, Rechavia E, Strasberg B, Agmon J: Ischemic ST segment depression in leads V2-V3 as the presenting electrocardiographic feature of posterolateral wall myocardial infarction. *Am Heart J* 113:1085–1090, 1987.

20. O'Keefe JH Jr, Sayed-Taha K, Gibson W, Christian TF, Bateman TM, Gibbons RJ: Do patients with left circumflex coronary artery-related acute myocardial infarction without ST-segment elevation benefit from reperfusion therapy? *Am J Cardiol* 75:718–720, 1995.

21. Schaer GL, Spaccavento LJ, Browne KF, Krueger KA, Gibbons RJ: A randomized double-blind, placebo-controlled trial of adjunctive therapy with RheothRx® injection (poloxamer 188) in patients receiving thrombolytic therapy for acute myocardial infarction (abstr). *J Am Coll Cardiol* Feb; Special Issue:344A, 1994.

22. Gruppo Italiano per lo Studio della Streptochinasi nell'Infarto Miocardio (GISSI): Long-term effects of intravenous thrombolysis in acute myocardial infarction: final report of the GISSI study. *Lancet* 2:871–874, 1987.

23. Krucoff MW, Green CE, Satler FL, et al: Noninvasive detection of coronary artery patency using continuous ST-segment monitoring. *Am J Cardiol* 57:916–922, 1986.

24. Krucoff MW, Croll MA, Pope JE, et al: Continuous 12-lead ST-segment recovery analysis in the TAMI 7 study. Performance of a noninvasive method for real-time detection of failed myocardial reperfusion. *Circulation* 88:437–446, 1993.

25. Fesmire FM, Wharton DR, Calhoun FB: Instability of ST segments in the early stages of acute myocardial infarction in patients undergoing continuous 12-lead ECG monitoring. *Am J Emerg Med* 13:158–163, 1995.

26. Murdock RH Jr, Chu A, Grubb M, Cobb FR: Effects of reestablishing blood flow

on extent of myocardial infarction in conscious dogs. *Am J Physiol* 249:H783–H791, 1985.

27. Christian TF, Schwartz RS, Gibbons RJ: Determinants of infarct size in reperfusion therapy for acute myocardial infarction. *Circulation* 86:81–90, 1992.

28. Christian TF, Gibbons RJ, Clements IP, Berger PB, Selvester RH, Wagner GS: Estimates of myocardium at risk and collateral flow in acute myocardial infarction using electrocardiographic indexes with comparison to radionuclide and angiographic measures. *J Am Coll Cardiol* 26:388–393, 1995.

29. Christian TF, Clements IP, Gibbons RJ: Noninvasive identification of myocardium at risk in patients with acute myocardial infarction and nondiagnostic electrocardiograms with technetium-99m-sestamibi. *Circulation* 83:1615–1620, 1991.

30. Fesmire FM: ECG diagnosis of acute myocardial infarction in the presence of left bundle-branch block in patients undergoing continuous ECG monitoring. *Ann Emerg Med* 26:69–82, 1995.

31. Maynard C, Litwin PE, Martin JS, Weaver WD: Gender differences in the treatment and outcome of acute myocardial infarction. Results from the Myocardial Infarction Triage and Intervention Registry. *Arch Intern Med* 152;972–976, 1992.

32. Dellborg M, Herlitz J, Emanuelsson H, Swedberg K: ECG changes during myocardial ischemia. Differences between men and women. *J Electrocardiol* 27(suppl): 42–45, 1994.

33. Raitt MH, Litwin PF, Martin JS, Weaver WD: ECG findings in acute myocardial infarction. Are there sex-related differences? *J Electrocardiol* 28:13–16, 1995.

11

Prognostic Indicators in the Initial Electrocardiogram During Acute Myocardial Infarction

Galen S. Wagner, MD

In 1983, at the very core of the prethrombolytic era, I wrote, "One should be certain that the patient with acute substernal chest pain receives coronary care, including single-lead-ECG (electrocardiographic) monitoring before a diagnostic 12-lead ECG is obtained. Information obtained from this single monitoring lead may be used to make optimal therapeutic decisions regarding the management of arrhythmias. Observation of the 12-lead ECGs allows the identification of either nontransmural (ST-segment depression or T-wave inversion) or transmural (ST-segment elevation, depression in the right precordial leads) ischemia. The epicardial-injury pattern permits localization of the area of myocardium in which transmural ischemia is present. Studies are now in progress to determine whether or not quantification of these ST-segment changes can indicate the amount of ischemic myocardium and, thereby, provide the basis for evaluation of interventions aimed at limiting myocardial infarct size."[1] Since that time, the thrombolytic era of coronary care has emerged, and many studies have been performed to identify the quantitative ECG criteria most capable of providing diagnostic and prognostic information.

It is helpful to understand the relationship between the left and right ventricular myocardium and the 12 standard body surface ECG leads. Figure 1A shows a frontal plane magnetic resonance image with the orderly sequenced limb leads oriented according to Einthoven's tri-

From: Clements, IP (ed). *The Electrocardiogram in Acute Myocardial Infarction.* Armonk, NY: Futura Publishing Company, Inc. © Mayo Foundation 1998.

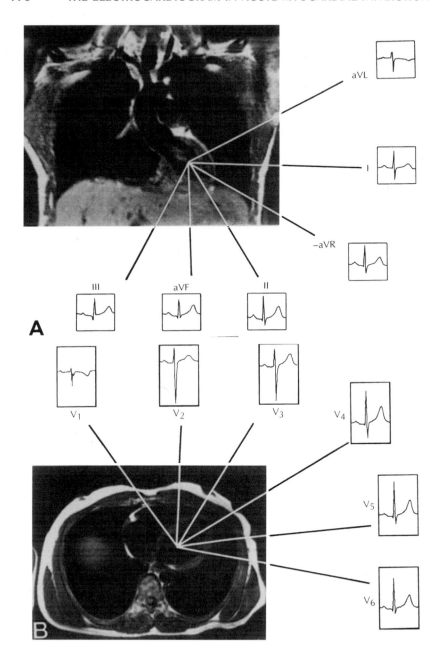

angle. Note that lead -aVR is positioned through the left ventricular apex.[2]

The horizontal plane is displayed in Figure 1B, with the positions of the six pericardial leads indicated. Note that lead V_6 in the midaxillary line overlies the posterior aspect of the left ventricular apex.

The typical distribution of the three major coronary arteries over the epicardial surface of the left ventricle is shown in a Mercator projection in Figure 2A. This specific quadrant subdivision, dividing the left ventricle circumferentially into four walls, has the advantage of dividing the septum along a line generally separating the perfusion beds of the septal perforating branches of the left anterior descending and the posterior descending coronary arteries. The inferior portion of the septum is included in the inferior wall. As indicated in the figure, the posterior descending artery is usually a branch of the right coronary artery, except when it forms the distal portion of a dominant left circumflex artery. The inferior apical segment and all three subdivisions of the anteroseptal and anterosuperior walls are supplied by the left anterior descending artery, except for the basal anterosuperior segment, which has a dual blood supply from the left circumflex artery. The posterolateral wall is supplied from the left circumflex artery, including some of its apical segment, which usually has a dual blood supply from the distal left anterior descending artery. The basal and middle segments of the inferior wall are supplied by the posterior descending artery.[2]

The regional distribution of myocardial infarcts in relation to their culprit coronary arteries is shown in the same Mercator projection in Figure 2B. The percentages indicate the number of patients in whom infarcts extend into that area of the left ventricle. For example, 9% of patients have infarcts limited to the area indicated in the apical sector of quadrant I and minimally into the other quadrants. In 13% of patients, infarcts extend farther into the middle sector of quadrant I and more of the apical sectors of the other three quadrants.

It is important to note that the majority of infarcts localize in the distal distribution of the vascular bed of the area at risk and involve less than one half of the potential risk area. Because of the smaller risk

---

Figure 1. Relationship between the left and right ventricular myocardium and the 12 body surface leads. **A.** Frontal plane magnetic resonance image with the orderly sequenced limb leads oriented according to Einthoven's triangle. Note that lead -aVR is positioned through the left ventricular apex. **B.** The horizontal plane (viewed from below) is displayed with the positions of the six precordial leads indicated. Note that the lead V_6 in the midaxillary line overlies the posterior aspect of the left ventricular apex. (Reproduced with permission from Anderson ST, Pahlm O, Selvester RH, et al: Panoramic display of the orderly sequenced 12-lead ECG. *J Electrocardiol* 27: 347–352, 1994.)

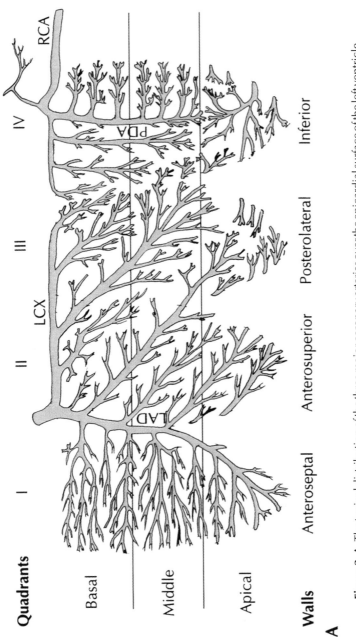

Figure 2. A. The typical distribution of the three major coronary arteries over the epicardial surface of the left ventricle (LV) is shown in a Mercator projection. This specific quadrant subdivision (I–IV) divides the LV circumferentially into four walls. It has the advantage of dividing the septum along a line generally separating the perfusion beds of the septal perforator branches of the left anterior descending (LAD) and the posterior descending (PDA) coronary arteries. The inferior portion of the septum is included in the inferior wall. As indicated here, the PDA is usually a branch of the right coronary artery (RCA) except when supplied by a dominant left circumflex (LCX) artery. The inferior apical segment and all three subdivisions of the anteroseptal and anterosuperior walls are supplied by the LAD, except for the basal anterosuperior segment, which has a dual blood supply from the LCX. The posterolateral wall is supplied from the LCX, including some of its apical segment, which usually has a dual blood supply from the distal LAD. The inferior wall is supplied by the RCA through its PDA and distal branches.

A

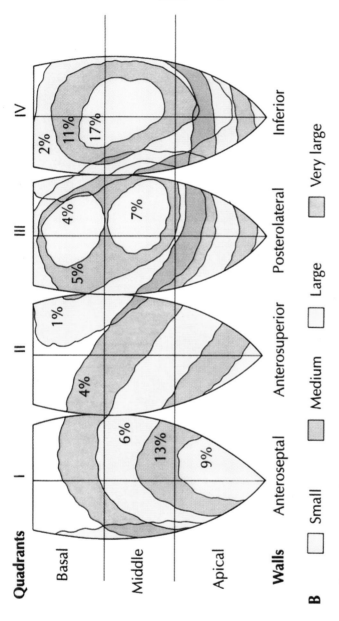

Figure 2. *(Continued)* **B.** The regional distribution of 80% of single infarcts in relation to their coronary arteries is shown in the same Mercator projection. The percentages indicate the numbers of patients in whom infarcts extend into that area of the LV. For example, 9% of patients have infarcts limited to the area indicated in the apical sector of quadrant I, and minimally into the other quadrants. In 13%, infarcts extend farther into the middle sector of quadrant I and more of the apical sectors of the other three quadrants. The 20% of patients who have multiple infarcts are not shown. It is important to note that the majority of infarcts localize in the distal distribution of the vascular bed of the area at risk and involve less than half of the potential risk area. Because of the smaller risk areas, both inferior and posterior infarcts tend to be small except in patients with a dominant LCX system. Large to very large infarcts involving more than 25% of the LV with ejection fractions below 40% and severe ventricular dysfunction occur in the anterior location in 10% of this group of single infarcts but are posterior and inferior in only 1% and 2%, respectively. (Reproduced with permission from Reference 2.)

areas, both inferior and posterior infarcts tend to be small, except in patients with a dominant left circumflex artery system. Large to very large infarcts involving more than 25% of the left ventricle, with ejection fractions less than 40% and severe ventricular dysfunction, occur in 10% of patients who have a single infarct in the anterior location. When the single infarct is posterior or inferior, such a large infarct occurs in only 1% and 2% of patients, respectively.[2]

It is helpful clinically to determine which leads best indicate the transmural ischemia produced by occlusion of the major coronary arteries. Figure 3 shows median ST-segment deviation for each lead and total median ST-segment deviation in the anterior and inferior locations on the admission ECGs of patients in the Duke Cardiovascular Data Bank during the 1970s.[3] If only two leads are considered, III and V_2 provide the most information about epicardial injury in both locations. The amount of ST-segment elevation on the initial ECG has been shown to correlate with the final infarct size when no thrombolytic therapy is given.[4] Table 1 shows that the number of leads with ST-segment elevation correlates best for the anterior location and the total amount of elevation correlates best for the inferior location.

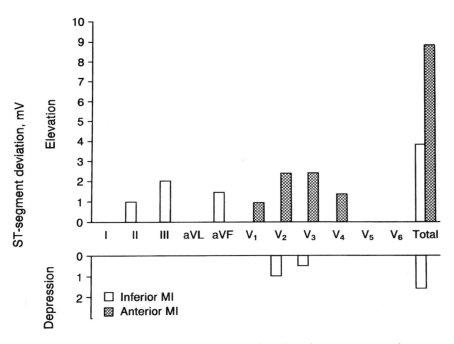

Figure 3. Median ST deviation for each lead and total median ST-segment deviation in each infarct group. MI = myocardial infarction. (Reproduced with permission from Reference 3.)

Table 1
Correlation of Admission ST-Segment Deviation With Pre-Discharge AMI Size

AMI Location	ST Variables	r
Anterior	Number of leads with ST-segment elevation	0.72
	ΣST-segment elevation all leads	0.52
	ΣST-segment elevation V_1 through V_3	0.38
	ΣST-segment elevation V_1 through V_6	0.48
	ΣST-segment elevation V_1 through V_3 I, aVL	0.46
Inferior	Number of leads with ST-segment elevation	0.50
	ΣST-segment elevation all leads	0.61
	ΣST-segment elevation all leads + ΣST-segment depression V_1 through V_3	0.60
	ΣST-segment elevation II, III, aVF	0.61
	ΣST-segment elevation II, III, aVF + ΣST-segment depression V_1 through V_3	0.59

AMI = acute myocardial infarction.
(Reproduced with permission from Reference 4.)

Weighted formulas were derived by Aldrich et al[4] and Clemmensen et al[5] from these relationships to predict the final infarct (MI) size from the amount of initial ST-segment elevation (ST↑):

Anterior: % MI size = 3 [1.5 (no. of leads with (ST↑) − 0.4]
Inferior: % MI size = 3 [0.6 (ΣST↑ II, III, aVF) + 2.0]

Figure 4 shows the correlations between the sum of ST-segment elevation and both global (A) and regional (B) left ventricular function in patients with and without coronary artery reperfusion after thrombolytic therapy. There are poor correlations in reperfused patients because the ST-segment elevation has already begun to resolve, while mechanical stunning delays the increase in left ventricular ejection fraction and decrease in regional hypocontractility.[6]

The "Aldrich" method for estimating the final infarct size from the admission ECG is applied to inferior and anterior infarctions in Figure 5.[7] The percent-predicted infarction for the prehospital ECG and the emergency room ECG is calculated below the corresponding recording. The variation in percent-predicted infarction is calculated below the emergency room ECG. In the example of an inferior myocardial infarction, the estimated salvage is 5%. In contrast, the final size in the example of an anterior myocardial infarction exceeds that predicted by 5%.

Twelve-lead ECGs from patients with acute anterior and inferior myocardial infarctions who received thrombolytic therapy are shown in Figure 6. The calculation of the initial ST-predicted infarct size, the final QRS-estimated infarct size, and the percent difference are also

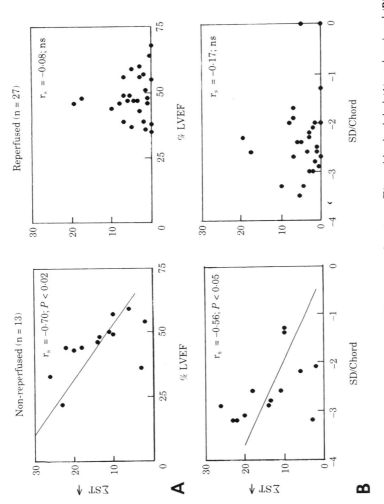

Figure 4. Correlations between the sum of ST-segment elevations (∑↑) and both global (**A**) and regional (**B**) left ventricular function in patients with and without coronary artery reperfusion following thrombolytic therapy. LVEF = left ventricular ejection fraction; SD = standard deviation. (Reproduced with permission from Reference 6.)

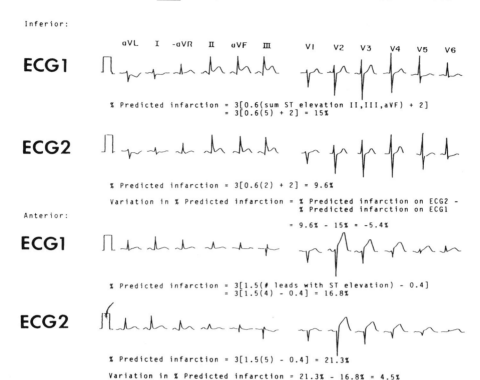

Figure 5. The method is applied to inferior and anterior infarct locations. The percent-predicted infarction for the prehospital ECG (ECG1) and the emergency room ECG (ECG2) is calculated below the corresponding ECG. The variation in percent-predicted infarction is calculated below ECG2. (Reproduced with permission from Reference 7.)

shown. Note the absence of extensive Q-wave development, despite marked ST-segment deviation on the admission ECG indicting extensive myocardial salvage.

Each patient's percent change from the initial ST-predicated infarct size to the final QRS-estimated infarct size in a control group ($n = 40$) and a group treated with streptokinase ($n = 33$) is depicted in Figure 7.[8] This ECG technique demonstrates considerable myocardial salvage following streptokinase.

Achievement of salvage requires early and complete restoration of coronary blood flow. When patients are grouped according to their initial Thrombolysis in Myocardial Infarction (TIMI) grade flow, only those with TIMI grade 3 flow on their admission angiogram showed both ECG and ventriculographic evidence of salvage by the time of hospital

I   II   III   aVR   aVL   aVF   V₁   V₂   V₃   V₄   V₅   V₆

Initial ST-predicted MI size = 3[1.5(no. of leads with ST↑) − 0.4]
  = 3[1.5(6) − 0.4]
  = 26%

Final QRS-estimated MI size = 3[QRS score]
  = 3[1]
  = 3%

$$\text{Percent difference} = 100 \times \frac{\text{Final QRS-estimated MI size} - \text{Initial ST-predicted MI size}}{\text{Initial ST-predicted MI size}}$$

$$= 100 \times \frac{3 - 26}{26}$$

$$= -88\%$$

A

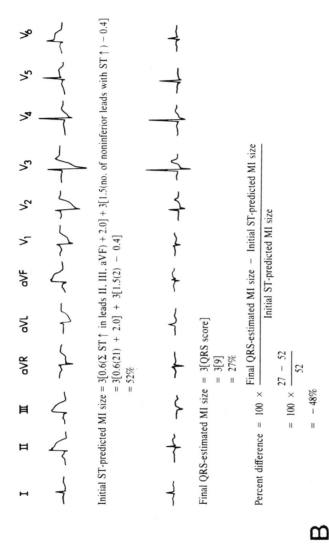

Figure 6. Twelve-lead ECG of a patient with, **A**, acute anterior myocardial infarction (MI) and, **B**, acute inferior MI. Calculation of initial ST-predicted infarct size, final QRS-estimated infarct size, and percent difference is shown. Σ = sum; ↑ = elevation. (Reproduced with permission from Reference 8.)

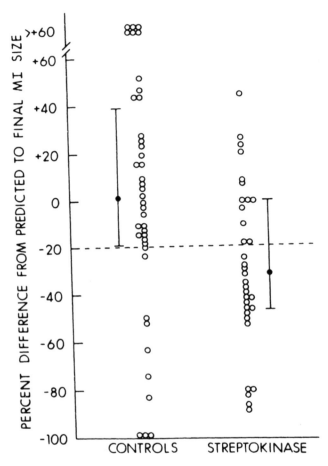

Figure 7. Each patient's (**open circles**) percent change from initial ST-predicted myocardial infarct (MI) size to final QRS-estimated infarct size in the control group ($n =$
40) and the streptokinase group ($n = 33$). **Filled circles** = the median; **bars** = the
25th and 75th percentile levels for each group. **Broken line** at the 25th percentile
level for the control group, the proposed threshold for detection of myocardial salvage. Salvage is attributed to patients with a difference from predicted to final infarct
size on or below this line. (Reproduced with permission from Reference 8.)

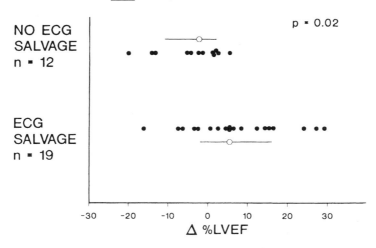

Figure 8. In-hospital change in global left ventricular ejection fraction (Δ % LVEF) in patients without (NO ECG SALVAGE) and in those with (ECG SALVAGE) ECG evidence of myocardial salvage. **Open circles** and **bars** = the median value and interquartile range, respectively. (Reproduced with permission from Reference 9.)

dismissal.[9] A moderate correlation ($r = 0.53$) was present between ECG and venticulographic-estimated myocardial salvage after intravenous thrombolysis. Figure 8 compares the in-hospital change in global left ventricular ejection fraction in patients without and those with ECG evidence of myocardial salvage. There was a slight decrease in the mean left ventricular ejection fraction in the "no salvage" group, but about a 5% increase in the "salvage" group.[9]

When the myocardium is reperfused after brief periods of occlusion in Prinzmetal's angina or angioplasty balloon occlusion, complete ST-segment resolution occurs almost immediately. However, when the occlusion has persisted during the early hours of an acute myocardial infarction, the myocardial reperfusion may be accompanied by much less than a rapid, complete disappearance of the ST-segment injury current. A study by Clemmensen et al[10] examined the sensitivity and specificity of various amounts of ST-segment changes for indicating angiographically documented reperfusion (Figure 9). Complete ST-segment resolution was associated with 100% specificity but only 15% sensitivity, whereas only 20% ST-segment resolution achieved approximately 80% levels of both specificity and sensitivity.

An accurate clinical evaluation of myocardial reperfusion requires both ECG and biochemical monitoring.[11] The serial changes produced by intracoronary thrombolysis in summated ST-segment elevation and serum myoglobin are presented in Figure 10. The time period from 60 minutes before until 90 minutes after angiographically documented reperfusion is indicated for three representative patients. In patient A,

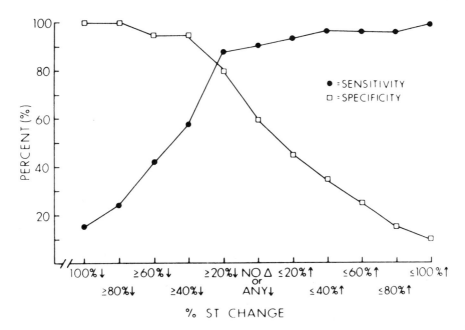

Figure 9. Spectra of sensitivities and specificities per % ST change in ST-segment elevation for identifying patients with myocardial reperfusion via a patent coronary artery. Values of sensitivity and specificity are given for each level of % ST change. For example, a % ST change of ≥20% decrease (↓) had a sensitivity of 88% and a specificity of 80% for identifying patients with reperfusion. (Reproduced with permission from Reference 10.)

there is a rapid decrease in ST-segment elevation and an increase in myoglobin. However, in patient B, the rapid decrease in ST-segment elevation is not accompanied by any increase in myoglobin, and in patient C, the increase in myoglobin is not accompanied by any decrease in ST-segment elevation. The clinical conclusion for patient B is that reperfusion occurred before infarction had occurred and, thus, no myoglobin had escaped from the cells. Conversely, in patient C, the reperfusion occurred so late that it did not reverse the injury current.

The myocardium at risk (Aldrich score) on admission and final myocardial infarct size (thallium) for patients receiving thrombolytic therapy at various time intervals after the onset of symptoms are compared in Figure 11.[12] The duration of symptoms before therapy was a significant predictor of final infarct size ($P < 0.0001$). Indeed, the final infarct size of patients receiving treatment more than 4 hours after the onset of symptoms and those who never received thrombolytic therapy was not different. Thus, the time until treatment is the primary determi-

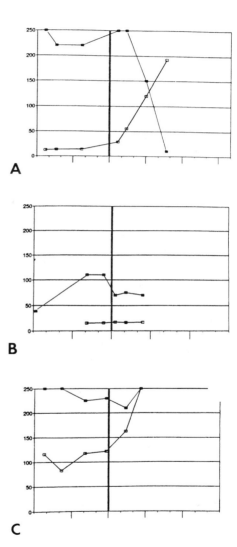

Figure 10. Serial changes produced by intracoronary thrombolysis (**solid vertical line**) in summated ST-segment elevation (■) in mV × 100 and serum myoglobin (□) in μg/L. The time, including 60 minutes before and 90 minutes after graphically documented reperfusion, is indicated in 10-minute intervals on the abscissa. **A.** There is a rapid decrease in ST-segment elevation and an increase in myoglobin. **B.** The rapid decrease in ST-segment elevation is not accompanied by an increase in myoglobin. **C.** The increase in myoglobin is not accompanied by any decrease in ST-segment elevation. (Reproduced with permission from Reference 11.)

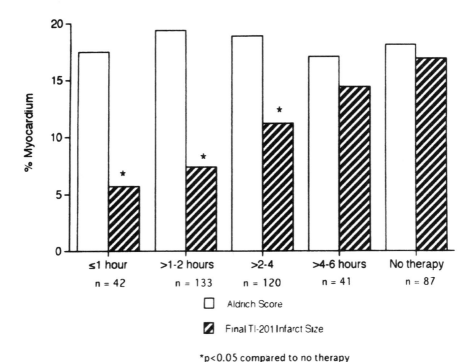

Figure 11. Estimated myocardium at risk (Aldrich score) and final myocardial infarct size, expressed as a percent of the myocardium, for patients with acute myocardial infarction treated with thrombolytic therapy at various time intervals after the onset of symptoms and for patients who did not receive thrombolytic therapy. Duration of symptoms before therapy was a significant predictor of final infarct size ($P < 0.0001$ by ANOVA). There was no difference in final infarct size between patients treated more than 4 hours after symptom onset and those who did not receive thrombolytic therapy. n = the number of patients from which the determinations were calculated. (Reproduced with permission from Reference 12.)

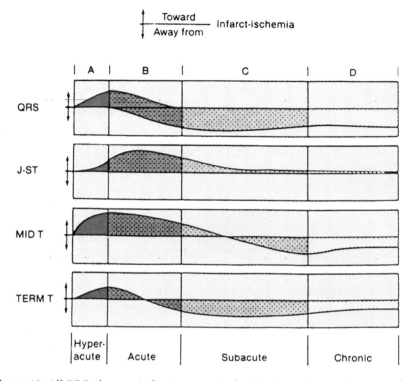

Figure 12. All ECG changes indicating ventricular depolarization and repolarization undergo sequential changes during the four phases of acute myocardial infarction: **A** = hyperacute; **B** = early acute and late acute; **C** = subacute; and **D** = chronic. ↑ = displacement of the electrical potential toward, and ↓ = away from the involved area of the heart. (Reproduced with permission from Reference 13.)

nant of success of reperfusion, and consideration of both ECG and biochemical changes provides clinical perspective.

All of the ECG changes that indicate ventricular depolarization and repolarization abnormalities undergo sequential changes during the minutes to hours after acute myocardial infarction. The four sequential phases that occur (hyperacute, acute, subacute, and chronic) are illustrated in Figure 12.[13]

Aspects of the ECG other than the ST segment may be altered during acute transmural ischemia.[14] The QRS complex undergoes change even before the onset of infarction. The QRS changes produced by the injury current are shown in Figure 13. On the "control" ECG obtained before balloon occlusion, the PR and ST segments can be used interchangeably as the baseline for the determination of waveform amplitudes. However, during occlusion, the terminal portion of the QRS is moved upward in association with the injury current. If the PR-segment baseline is used for determining waveform amplitudes, no S wave would be identified. The great variation in QRS changes during different periods of acute transmural ischemia is illustrated in Figure 14. Although the extent of ST-segment elevation is similar, a much greater QRS change occurred during inflation 1 than during inflation 3.[14]

Such QRS changes, beyond those related to the ST-segment deviation, most likely are caused by ischemia-induced intramyocardial conduction delay. Quantification of the QRS changes observed on the admission ECG may augment information available from the ST segment alone for clinical estimation of both the extent and potential reversibility of acute transmural ischemia.

Changes in the T wave also occur during the early minutes after acute transmural ischemia. Because these involve only T-wave magnitude rather than direction, it is necessary to be aware of the normal magnitudes in the various leads.[15] The marked differences in normal

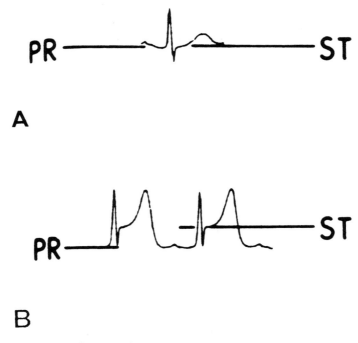

Figure 13. A. "Control" ECG. The PR and ST segments can be used interchangeably as the baseline for determination of waveform amplitudes. **B.** "Ischemic" ECG. The PR-segment baseline versus the shifted J-ST-segment baseline is used for determination of waveform amplitudes. (Reproduced with permission from Reference 14.)

CONTROL

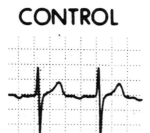

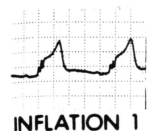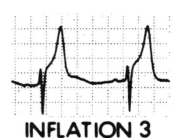

INFLATION 1   INFLATION 3

Figure 14. Lead V$_2$ ECGs taken during angioplasty in a patient illustrate the great variation in QRS change from inflation 1 to inflation 3, although the extent of ST-segment elevation is similar. A "periischemic block" was probably present during inflation 1 but absent during inflation 3. (Reproduced with permission from Reference 14.)

amplitudes of T waves in the various leads are shown in Figure 15. It might be most helpful to express T-wave changes as "excess T-wave amplitude" when quantifying the abnormality in a patient.

This chapter has presented data from recent studies documenting new uses for the standard ECG in evaluating patients with acute myocardial ischemia and infarction. Quantitative evaluation of ST-segment deviation and alterations in QRS complexes and T waves provides measures of the acuteness of the event, the severity of the ischemia, the completeness of reperfusion, and even the extent of salvage attained. Future studies may well provide more accurate methods for considering the relative changes in these various standard ECG variables and also determine whether consideration of additional leads, signal-averaged analysis, or vectorcardiographic methods (or a combination of these) will provide even further clinical usefulness.

In contrast to my 1983 statement, I can now conclude in 1996: One should be certain that the patient with acute substernal chest pain receives coronary care, including continuous multilead ECG monitoring and frequent sampling of biochemical markers such as myoglobin.

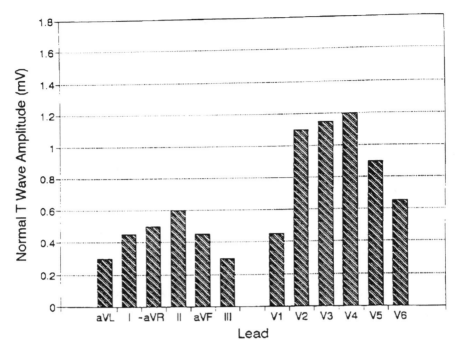

Figure 15. Distribution of the normal T-wave amplitude (mV) according to the ECG lead for the Duke University Medical Center and Bowman Gray School of Medicine populations combined (*n* = 1,935). (Reproduced with permission from Reference 15.)

References

1. Wagner GS, Corsa A, Hindman N: Prognostic indicators in the initial electrocardiogram during acute myocardial infarction. *Pract Cardiol* 9:198–217, 1983.
2. Wagner GS, Selvester RH: Part I: Clinical electrocardiography for quantification of myocardial infarction. In: Braunwald E (ed): *Atlas of Heart Diseases. Vol. 5. Chronic Ischemic Heart Disease.* St. Louis: Mosby-Year Book; 6.1–6.12, 1995.
3. Aldrich HR, Hindman NB, Hinohara T, et al: Identification of the optimal electrocardiographic leads for detecting acute epicardial injury in acute myocardial infarction. *Am J Cardiol* 59:20–23, 1987.
4. Aldrich HR, Wagner NB, Boswick J, et al: Use of initial ST-segment deviation for prediction of final electrocardiographic size of acute myocardial infarcts. *Am J Cardiol* 61:749–753, 1988.
5. Clemmensen P, Grande P, Aldrich HR, Wagner GS: Evaluation of formulas for estimating the final size of acute myocardial infarcts from quantitative ST-segment elevation on the initial standard 12-lead ECG. *J Electrocardiol* 24:77–83, 1991.
6. Clemmensen P, Ohman EM, Sevilla DC, et al: Impact of infarct artery patency

on the relationship between electrocardiographic and ventriculographic evidence of acute myocardial ischaemia. *Eur Heart J* 15:1356–1361, 1994.

7. Wilkins ML, Anderson ST, Pryor AD, Weaver WD, Wagner GS: Variability of acute ST-segment predicted myocardial infarct size in the absence of thrombolytic therapy. *Am J Cardiol* 74:174–177, 1994.

8. Clemmensen P, Grande P, Saunamaki K, et al: Effect of intravenous streptokinase on the relation between initial ST-predicted size and final QRS-estimated size of acute myocardial infarcts. *J Am Coll Cardiol* 16:1252–1257, 1990.

9. Clemmensen P, Ohman EM, Sevilla DC, et al: Importance of early and complete reperfusion to achieve myocardial salvage after thrombolysis in acute myocardial infarction. *Am J Cardiol* 70:1391–1396, 1992.

10. Clemmensen P, Ohman EM, Sevilla DC, et al: Changes in standard electrocardiographic ST-segment elevation predictive of successful reperfusion in acute myocardial infarction. *Am J Cardiol* 66:1407–1411, 1990.

11. Ohman EM, Christenson R, Clemmensen P, Wagner GS: Myocardial salvage after reperfusion. Observations from analysis of serial electrocardiographic and biochemical indices. *J Electrocardiol* 25(suppl):10–14, 1992.

12. Raitt MH, Maynard C, Wagner GS, Cerqueira MD, Selvester RH, Weaver WD: Relationship between symptom duration before thrombolytic therapy and final myocardial infarct size. *Circulation* 93:48–53, 1996.

13. Wagner NB, Wagner GS: ECG criteria guiding the selection of MI patients for thrombolytic therapy. *Prim Cardiol* 15 no. 12:28–38, 1989.

14. Wagner NB, Sevilla DC, Krucoff MW, et al: Transient alterations of the QRS complex and ST segment during percutaneous transluminal balloon angioplasty of the left anterior descending coronary artery. *Am J Cardiol* 623:1038–1042, 1988.

15. Gambill CL, Wilkins ML, Haisty WK Jr, et al: T wave amplitudes in normal populations. Variation with ECG lead, sex, and age. *J Electrocardiol* 28:191–197, 1995.

12

Atypical Electrocardiographic Patterns in Acute Myocardial Infarction

Ian P. Clements, MD

Atypical ECG Markers of Infarction

The electrocardiographic (ECG) marker typical for evolving acute myocardial infarction is ST-segment elevation. The leads in which ST-segment elevation occur mark the distribution of the initial transmural myocardial ischemia and localize the infarct-related artery to the left anterior descending, circumflex, or right coronary artery distribution. Usually, leads that show ST-segment elevation develop the classic Q waves of transmural myocardial infarction. However, there are many patients with evolving infarction in which this typical pattern is not followed.[1] In fact, typical ST-segment elevation and Q-wave myocardial infarction occur in 50% or fewer patients. This chapter discusses some of the atypical ECG patterns of acute myocardial infarction.

Normal Electrocardiogram in Myocardial Infarction

The ECG may appear normal in myocardial infarction. This is relatively rare, but it has been noted to occur in 10% to 20% of patients early in myocardial infarction.[2,3] Thus, it is important to take clinical features such as chest pain features and physical examination findings into ac-

From: Clements, IP (ed). *The Electrocardiogram in Acute Myocardial Infarction.* Armonk, NY: Futura Publishing Company, Inc. © Mayo Foundation 1998.

count in these circumstances; otherwise, patients in whom myocardial infarction will evolve may not be admitted for monitoring and pain control. It is possible that noninvasive testing, including echocardiography and perfusion imaging, in these circumstances would detect myocardial ischemia.

ST-Segment Depression in Acute Myocardial Infarction

Patients with ST-segment depression have a high mortality, 16% to 19%,[4,5] that is not reduced by thrombolysis. Lee et al[6] studied a group of 136 consecutive patients with ST-segment depression admitted to the Coronary Care Unit in Aberdeen. Of these patients, 54% had confirmed infarction. Prior myocardial infarction was common in this population (54%), and the patients were elderly (mean age ± SD, 68 ± 12 yr). The 1-year mortality in this population was 35% for those not receiving thrombolysis and 24% in those who had thrombolysis. It is of note that for the 74 patients with confirmed infarction, the 1-year mortality was 31%, as compared with 19% for the 62 patients who did not have confirmed infarction.

One-year mortality was significantly less in patients with only 1 mm ST-segment depression (14%) than in those with 2 mm or more ST-segment depression (39%).

The number of leads with ST-segment depression was also a predictor of mortality. If only one or two leads were involved, 1-year mortality was 11%, in comparison with 30% if three or more leads were involved.

The extent and degree of ST-segment depression also predicted the likelihood of infarction. Patients who had confirmed infarction had more severe ($P < 0.001$) ST-segment depression (mean ± SD, 2.5 ± 1.5 mm) than those in whom infarction was excluded (1.4 ± 0.8). The patients with infarction had a greater number of leads involved (4.7 ± 1.8 vs 3.6 ± 1.7, $P < 0.001$).

Anterior ST-Segment Depression in Inferior Myocardial Infarction

The presence of anterior ST-segment depression in acute inferior myocardial infarction has been studied for many years (Figure 1).[7–9] The anterior ST-depression in these circumstances has been termed "reciprocal"—that is, it is the mirror image of the ST-segment elevation in the inferior leads.

Other potential causes for anterior ST-segment depression are anterior ischemia and more extensive myocardial infarction.

In 1985, Lew et al[10] studied 61 patients who had isolated acute

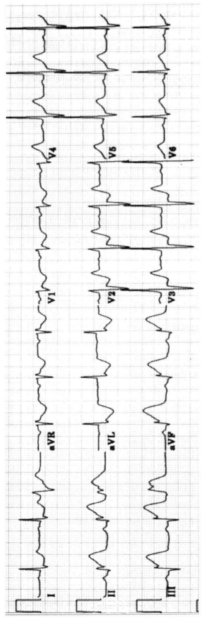

Figure 1. Anterior ST-segment depression in a patient with inferior infarction.

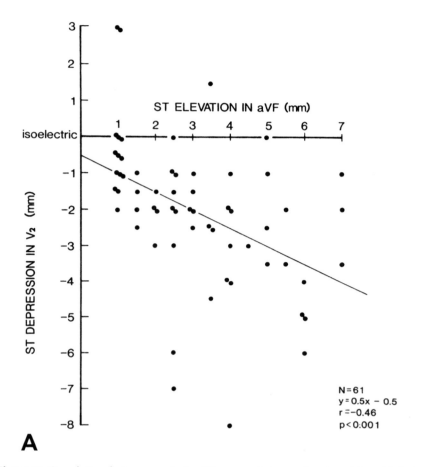

Figure 2. Correlation between anterior ST-segment depression (y-axis) and inferior ST-elevation (x-axis) in patients with acute inferior myocardial infarction. **A.** All patients. **B.** Patients without right ventricular or lateral wall involvement. (Reproduced with permission from Reference 10.)

inferior infarction. From the ECGs, these authors determined right ventricular and lateral wall involvement. They argued that these additional areas of myocardial involvement in inferior infarction distorted the relationship between anterior ST-segment depression and inferior ST-segment elevation. These latter two factors had a low correlation of -0.46 if all 61 patients (Figure 2A) were considered, but the correlation was better ($r = -0.89$) in patients without right ventricular and lateral wall involvement (Figure 2B).

Right ventricular involvement was found to be associated with re-

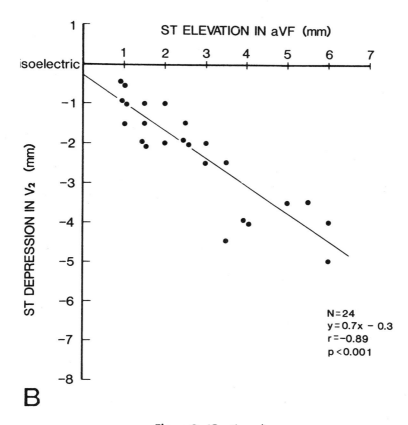

Figure 2. *(Continued)*

duced anterior ST-segment depression, whereas lateral wall involvement was associated with greater ST-segment depression in the anterior leads. Lew et al[10] emphasized that right ventricular and lateral wall involvement have independent and opposite effects on the magnitude of precordial ST-segment depression. It is of note that no patient in this study had an occluded left anterior descending coronary artery. Also, of the 40 patients who underwent thallium-201 imaging, none had proximal anterior perfusion abnormality; 13 patients had a mild perfusion abnormality in the distal anterior wall.

Other workers have found that anterior ST-segment depression in acute inferior infarction is associated with a larger area of infarction and a worse long-term prognosis (Figure 3).[11] Ruddy et al[12] found that anterior ST-segment depression in acute inferior infarction was associated with greater wall motion and perfusion abnormality in the inferior and posterolateral segments, but not in the anterior segment and septal wall motion and perfusion abnormalities.

Gibelin et al[13] reported that anterior ST-segment depression in acute infarction was associated with greater myocardial necrosis and a greater incidence of significant disease of the left coronary system, with three-vessel coronary disease evident in 71% of patients with anterior ST-segment depression, as compared with 29% of those without anterior ST-segment depression. Other investigators have suggested that anterior ST-segment depression is a marker for left coronary artery disease in these circumstances.[14] However, other studies have failed to associate left coronary artery disease with anterior ST-segment depression.[9,15]

Anterior ST-segment depression has been studied recently in the setting of evolving inferior myocardial infarction using technetium Tc 99m sestamibi. It was confirmed that anterior ST-segment depression is associated with a more extensive area of inferior myocardium being at risk and with involvement of the posterolateral wall of the heart (Fig-

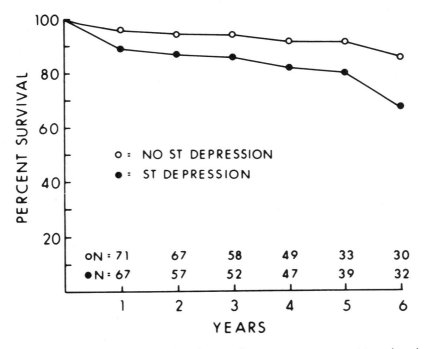

Figure 3. Survival of patients with inferior infarction over 6 years. Note that the presence of anterior ST-segment depression (**solid circles**) is associated with a worse survival than the absence of anterior ST-depression (**open circles**). (Reproduced with permission from Reference 11.)

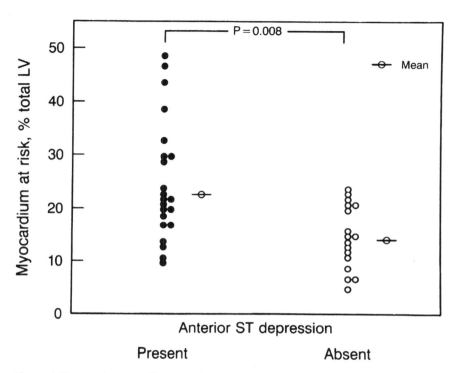

Figure 4. Extent of myocardium at risk in patients with or without anterior ST-segment depression in evolving acute inferior myocardial infarction. LV = left ventricle. (Reproduced with permission from Reference 16.)

ure 4).[16] Anterior perfusion abnormalities were not seen in these studies.

Precordial Mapping and ST-Segment Depression in Inferior Infarction

Walker et al[17] studied precordial body surface ECG maps in patients with inferior infarction and found that a large amount of ST-segment depression in the precordial map was associated with a higher mortality, more heart failure, and more arrhythmia. Also, the difference between ST-segment depression and elevation on the precordial map—if marked—was associated with a high mortality. In addition, a precordial map that showed predominantly ST-segment depression was a predictor of a higher hospital mortality.

Inferior ST-Segment Depression in Anterior Infarction

Inferior ST-segment depression in anterior infarction has been ascribed as reciprocal to ST-segment elevation in the anterior leads in anterior infarction and to possible ischemia at a distance (Figure 5). Studies in evolving myocardial infarction indicate that patients with anterior infarction and inferior ST-segment depression demonstrate extension of infarction into the lateral wall; ischemia in the inferior wall was not demonstrated.[18]

An interesting study by Lew et al[19] suggested that ST-segment depression in the inferior leads in anterior myocardial infarction was truly a reciprocal phenomenon. These workers showed that in anterior infarction, inferior ST-segment depression occurred when the distal portion of the occluded left anterior descending coronary artery did not supply the inferoapical surface of the heart. In contrast, when the occluded left anterior descending coronary artery supplied the inferoapical surface, the ST segment in the inferior leads tended to be isoelectric or elevated. These authors suggested that the latter situation reflected inferior transmural ischemia, nullifying or overwhelming the reciprocal effect on the ECG. This hypothesis was supported by the finding that, when anterior ST-segment elevation occurred in the absence of inferior ST-segment depression, perfusion imaging showed transmural ischemia extending from the anterior wall to the inferoapical region. In contrast, when inferior ST-segment depression was present, perfusion imaging showed normal perfusion of the inferior wall. In the former circumstance, the left anterior descending coronary artery ran beyond the apex inferiorly; in the latter circumstance, the artery was limited to the anterior wall of the heart.

Right Ventricular Infarction

The ECG can be used to identify right ventricular infarction. Cohn et al[20] identified ST-segment elevation in the right precordial leads as a marker for right ventricular infarction. Other workers have confirmed this finding, and several reviews of the ECG in right ventricular infarction are available.[21,22]

Lew et al[23] noted that right ventricular involvement was associated with a ratio of the ST-segment depression in V_2 of 50% or less of the magnitude of ST-segment elevation in aVF. These criteria had a 90% positive and a 32% negative predictive value for identifying right ventricular ischemia.

Right ventricular infarction usually occurs in combination with inferior myocardial infarction. Isolated right ventricular infarction is rare. Vermeersch et al[24] noted the ECG findings of ST-segment elevations in

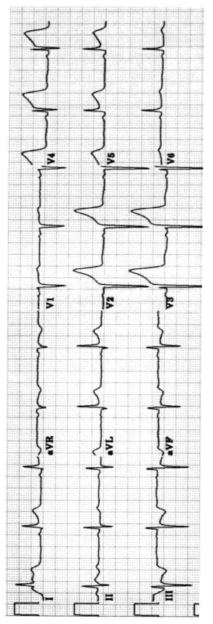

Figure 5. ECG showing ST-segment depression in the inferior leads in the setting of acute anterior myocardial infarction.

leads V_{4R} and aVR and leads V_1-V_4. These findings were associated with occlusion of a large right ventricular branch of the right coronary artery. This pattern has been noted by other workers.[25,26] An unusual pattern of ST-segment elevation in leads II, III, aVF, and V_1-V_3 consistent with right ventricular and inferior infarction are indicated in Figure 6.

Acute Myocardial Infarction in Left Bundle Branch Block

Traditionally, acute infarction has been difficult to diagnose in left bundle branch block. In the thrombolytic era, left bundle branch block was considered an exclusion to thrombolysis because it was believed that acute infarction could not be diagnosed definitely. However, the occurrence of left bundle branch block with clinical features of acute infarction should not be an exclusion to reperfusion strategies. It may indicate a large myocardial infarction. In fact, such patients may benefit most from reperfusion.

Under certain circumstances, Q waves on the ECG of a person with left bundle branch block indicate infarction. The presence of Q waves in the lateral chest leads is indicative of septal infarction.[27] Several other features on the ECG indicate acute myocardial infarction in left bundle branch block. Marked ST-segment elevation in the presence of left bundle branch block is a marker of acute infarction, particularly if present in the inferior leads and in I and aVL.[28]

Electrocardiographic Changes in Occlusion of the Circumflex Coronary Artery

Acute occlusion of the left circumflex coronary artery produces atypical ECG changes for acute transmural infarction. Commonly, occlusion of this vessel produces ST-segment depression. The occurrence of ST-segment depression of V_1-V_3 in the presence of symptoms of infarction is highly likely to be associated with occlusion of the circumflex coronary artery.[29,30] In addition, ST-segment elevation inferiorly and ST-segment depression anteriorly frequently reflect acute occlusion of this artery.[31]

Posterior infarction with ST-segment depression in V_1-V_3 and prominent R-wave voltage in the same leads most commonly is caused by acute occlusion of the circumflex coronary artery.

Posterior Myocardial Infarction

Boden et al[32] studied 50 patients with isolated ST-segment depression of 1 mm or more in two or more contiguous precordial leads (V_1-V_4).

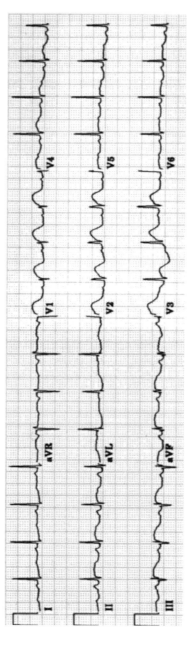

Figure 6. ECG of a patient with acute right ventricular infarction with associated inferior infarction. ST-segment elevation is present in leads II, III, aVF, and V_1-V_3.

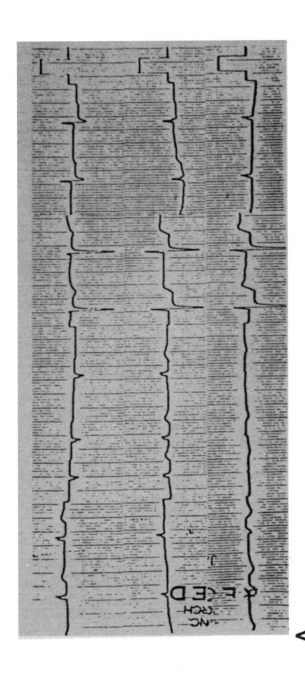

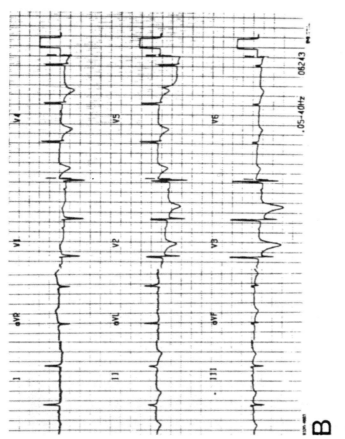

Figure 7. ECGs of two patients with anterior ST-segment depression in leads V_1-V_3. The ECGs are typical of: **A,** acute posterior infarction and, **B,** acute nontransmural anterior infarction. (Reproduced with permission from Reference 32.)

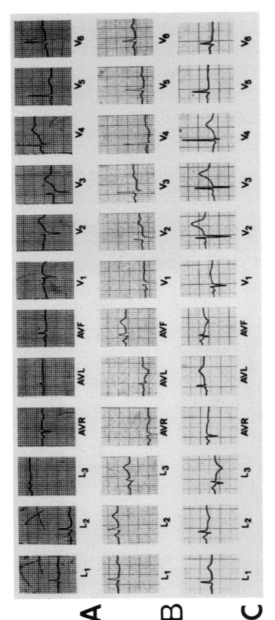

Figure 8. A-C. ECGs of patient with inferior myocardial infarction. The development of an inverted T wave in lead aVL with onset of chest pain (**B**) compared with an ECG taken some months earlier (**A**) suggests acute inferior myocardial infarction, despite the absence of significant ST-segment elevation in leads L$_2$, L$_3$, and aVF. **C.** The ECG 5 days after hospital admission shows new Q waves in L$_2$, L$_3$, and aVF, indicative of an evolved inferior myocardial infarction. (Reproduced with permission from Reference 34.)

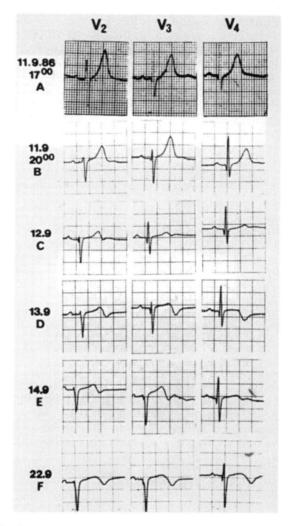

Figure 9. Peaked T-waves in anterior leads. Representative ECG tracing of evolving anterior wall myocardial infarction. **A.** During prolonged chest pain showing positive peaked T waves without ST-segment elevation. **B-F.** Gradual shortening of R waves and late appearance of Q waves. (Reproduced with permission from Reference 35.)

These patients were identified from 544 patients with non-Q-wave acute myocardial infarction in the multicenter Diltiazem Reinfarction Study. Of the 50 patients, 23 developed ECG evidence of posterior infarction (R wave ≥ 0.04 second in V_1 and an R:S ≥ 1 in V_2). The other 27 patients were considered to have had an anterior non–Q-wave infarction. It is of note that patients in whom a posterior infarction developed had greater ST-segment depression that tended to be horizontal and an upright T-wave; in comparison, patients with an anterior non–Q-wave myocardial infarction had a lesser degree of ST-segment depression that was downsloping and inverted T waves anteriorly (Figure 7).

Because patients with posterior infarction have a greater increase in creatine phosphokinase than patients with non–Q-wave infarction, they should be considered for thrombolytic therapy.

Prediction of an Isolated First Diagonal Branch Occlusion

Occlusion of the first diagonal branch of the left anterior descending coronary artery has been found to produce isolated ST-segment elevation in leads I and aVL.[33] If ST-segment elevation occurred in I and aVL and the precordial leads, then occlusion of the left anterior descending coronary artery was more likely.

Other Unusual ECG Features Suggestive of Infarction

Birnbaum et al[34] pointed out that ST-segment depression in aVL may be a sensitive marker for acute inferior infarction (Figure 8).

Peaked T waves in the anterior leads in the absence of ST-segment elevation in the clinical setting of acute myocardial infarction have been said to indicate total occlusion of the left anterior descending coronary artery with retrograde filling of the artery via collaterals (Figure 9).[35]

References

1. Rude RE, Poole WK, Muller JE, et al: Electrocardiographic and clinical criteria for recognition of acute myocardial infarction based on analysis of 3,697 patients. *Am J Cardiol* 52:936–942, 1983.
2. Cunningham SR, Dalzell GWN, Adgey AAJ: Initial electrocardiograms and outcome for patients seen by a mobile coronary care unit within four hours of the onset of suspected myocardial infarction (abstr). *Br Heart J* 59:628–629, 1988.
3. Slater DK, Hlatky MA, Mark DB, Harrell FE Jr, Pryor DB, Califf RM: Outcome in suspected acute myocardial infarction with normal or minimally abnormal admission electrocardiographic findings. *Am J Cardiol* 60:766–770, 1987.

4. Gruppo Italiano per lo Studio della Streptochinasi nell'Infarto Miocardico (GISSI): Effectiveness of intravenous thrombolytic treatment in acute myocardial infarction. *Lancet* 1:387–402, 1986.
5. ISIS-2 (Second International Study of Infarct Survival) Collaborative Group: Randomised trial of intravenous streptokinase, oral aspirin, both, or neither among 17,187 cases of suspected acute myocardial infarction: ISIS-2. *Lancet* 2: 349–360, 1988.
6. Lee HS, Cross SJ, Rawles JM, Jennings KP: Patients with suspected myocardial infarction who present with ST depression. *Lancet* 342:1204–1207, 1993.
7. Croft CH, Woodward W, Nicod P, et al: Clinical implications of anterior S-T segment depression in patients with acute inferior myocardial infarction. *Am J Cardiol* 50:428–436, 1982.
8. Shah PK, Pichler M, Berman DS, et al: Noninvasive identification of a high risk subset of patients with acute inferior myocardial infarction. *Am J Cardiol* 46: 915–921, 1980.
9. Gibson RS, Crampton RS, Watson DD, et al: Precordial ST-segment depression during acute inferior myocardial infarction: clinical, scintigraphic and angiographic correlations. *Circulation* 66:732–741, 1982.
10. Lew AS, Maddahi J, Shah PK, et al: Factors that determine the direction and magnitude of precordial ST-segment deviations during inferior wall acute myocardial infarction. *Am J Cardiol* 55:883–888, 1985.
11. Hlatky MA, Califf RM, Lee KL, Pryor DB, Wagner GS, Rosati RA: Prognostic significance of precordial ST-segment depression during inferior acute myocardial infarction. *Am J Cardiol* 55:325–329, 1985.
12. Ruddy TD, Yasuda T, Gold HK, et al: Anterior ST segment depression in acute inferior myocardial infarction as a marker of greater inferior, apical, and posterolateral damage. *Am Heart J* 112:1210–1216, 1986.
13. Gibelin P, Gilles B, Baudouy M, Guarino L, Morand P: Reciprocal ST segment changes in acute inferior myocardial infarction: clinical, haemodynamic and angiographic implications. *Eur Heart J* 7:133–139, 1986.
14. Salcedo JR, Baird MG, Chambers RJ, Beanlands DS: Significance of reciprocal ST-segment depression in anterior precordial leads in acute inferior myocardial infarction: concomitant left anterior descending coronary artery disease? *Am J Cardiol* 48:1003–1008, 1981.
15. Ferguson DW, Pandian N, Kioschos JM, Marcus ML, White CW: Angiographic evidence that reciprocal ST-segment depression during acute myocardial infarction does not indicate remote ischemia: analysis of 23 patients. *Am J Cardiol* 53:55–62, 1984.
16. Edmunds JJ, Gibbons RJ, Bresnahan JF, Clements IP: Significance of anterior ST depression in inferior wall acute myocardial infarction. *Am J Cardiol* 73: 143–148, 1994.
17. Walker SJ, Bell AJ, Loughhead MG, Lavercombe PS, Kilpatrick D: Spatial distribution and prognostic significance of ST segment potential determined by body surface mapping in patients with acute inferior myocardial infarction. *Circulation* 76:289–297, 1987.
18. Fletcher WO, Gibbons RJ, Clements IP: The relationship of inferior ST depression, lateral ST elevation, and left precordial ST elevation to myocardium at risk in acute anterior myocardial infarction. *Am Heart J* 126:526–535, 1993.
19. Lew AS, Hod H, Cercek B, Shah PK, Ganz W: Inferior ST segment changes during acute anterior myocardial infarction: a marker of the presence or absence of concomitant inferior wall ischemia. *J Am Coll Cardiol* 10:519–526, 1987.

20. Cohn JN, Guiha NH, Broder MI, Limas CJ: Right ventricular infarction. Clinical and hemodynamic features. *Am J Cardiol* 33:209–214, 1974.
21. Erhardt LR, Sjogren A, Wahlberg I: Single right-sided precordial lead in the diagnosis of right ventricular involvement in inferior myocardial infarction. *Am Heart J* 91:571–576, 1976.
22. Croft CH, Nicod P, Corbett JR, et al: Detection of acute right ventricular infarction by right precordial electrocardiography. *Am J Cardiol* 50:421–427, 1982.
23. Lew AS, Laramee P, Shah PK, Maddahi J, Peter T, Ganz W: Ratio of ST-segment depression in lead V2 to ST-segment elevation in lead aVF in evolving inferior acute myocardial infarction: an aid to the early recognition of right ventricular ischemia. *Am J Cardiol* 57:1047–1051, 1986.
24. Vermeersch PHMJ, TjonJoeGin RM, Plokker HWT, et al: Isolated acute occlusion of a large right ventricular branch of the right coronary artery: the only true "model" to study ECG changes in acute, isolated RV infarction. *Circulation* 88(suppl 1):I-306, 1993.
25. Geft IL, Shah PK, Rodriguez L, et al: ST elevations in leads V1 to V5 may be caused by right coronary artery occlusion and acute right ventricular infarction. *Am J Cardiol* 53:991–996, 1984.
26. Chou TC, Van der Bel-Kahn J, Allen J, Brockmeier L, Fowler NO: Electrocardiographic diagnosis of right ventricular infarction. *Am J Med* 70:1175–1180, 1981.
27. Horan LG, Flowers NC, Tolleson WJ, Thomas JR: The significance of diagnostic Q waves in the presence of bundle branch block. *Chest* 58:214–220, 1970.
28. Sgarbossa EB, Pinski SL, Barbagelata NA, et al: Electrocardiographic diagnosis of impending acute infarction in the presence of left bundle branch block (abstr). *Circulation* 90(suppl 4):I-444, 1994.
29. Bairey CN, Shah PK, Lew AS, Hulse S: Electrocardiographic differentiation of occlusion of the left circumflex versus the right coronary artery as a cause of inferior acute myocardial infarction. *Am J Cardiol* 60:456–459, 1987.
30. Blanke H, Cohen M, Schlueter GU, Karsch KR, Rentrop KP: Electrocardiographic and coronary arteriographic correlations during acute myocardial infarction. *Am J Cardiol* 54:249–255, 1984.
31. Huey BL, Beller GA, Kaiser DL, Gibson RS: A comprehensive analysis of myocardial infarction due to left circumflex artery occlusion: comparison with infarction due to right coronary artery and left anterior descending artery occlusion. *J Am Coll Cardiol* 12:1156–1166, 1988.
32. Boden WE, Kleiger RE, Gibson RS, et al: Electrocardiographic evolution of posterior acute myocardial infarction: importance of early precordial ST-segment depression. *Am J Cardiol* 59:782–787, 1987.
33. Iwasaki K, Kusachi S, Kita T, Taniguchi G: Prediction of isolated first diagonal branch occlusion by 12-lead electrocardiography: ST segment shift in leads I and aVL. *J Am Coll Cardiol* 23:1557–1561, 1994.
34. Birnbaum Y, Sclarovsky S, Mager A, Strasberg B, Rechavia E: ST segment depression in aVL: a sensititve marker for acute inferior myocardial infarction. *Eur Heart J* 14:4–7, 1993.
35. Sagie A, Sclarovsky S, Strasberg B, et al: Acute anterior wall myocardial infarction presenting with positive T waves and without ST segment shift. Electrocardiographic features and angiographic correlation. *Chest* 95:1211–1215, 1989.

13

Triage of Acute Infarction Using Prehospital Electrocardiograms

Stephen R. McMechan, MB, MRCP
Mark T. Harbinson, MB, MRCP
Shahid Hameed, MRCP
A. A. Jennifer Adgey, MD, FRCP, FACC

Introduction

The standard 12-lead electrocardiogram (ECG) is an indispensable tool in the assessment of patients with acute chest pain. The ECG is important in establishing the diagnosis of acute myocardial infarction, in giving some estimate of prognosis, and in assisting in the triage of patients with various chest pain syndromes. The main purpose in recording the ECG outside the hospital is to decrease the time delay for administering thrombolytic treatment to patients with definite myocardial infarction. In this chapter, we address the value and limitations of the 12-lead ECG in the prehospital setting and include examples of cases presenting to our cardiology unit.

The Importance of Early Detection of Acute Myocardial Infarction

The majority of deaths from myocardial infarction are sudden; they occur within 1 hour after the onset of symptoms and, thus, before the

From: Clements, IP (ed). *The Electrocardiogram in Acute Myocardial Infarction.*
Armonk, NY: Futura Publishing Company, Inc. © Mayo Foundation 1998.

patient reaches a hospital. Also, the effectiveness of thrombolytic therapy among patients with suspected acute myocardial infarction is maximal within 1 hour after the onset of symptoms. In the Gruppo Italiano per lo Studio Della Streptochinasi nell'Infarto Miocardico (GISSI)-1 trial[1] (initial report) for those receiving streptokinase within 1 hour after symptom onset, the in-hospital mortality rate was reduced by 47%. In the Second International Study of Infarct Survival (ISIS)-2 study,[2] among those receiving streptokinase plus aspirin within a similar time period, the 5-week vascular mortality rate was reduced by 56%.

The prehospital administration of thrombolytic therapy has achieved a significant decrease in the time to start treatment and, with earlier treatment, an associated decrease in infarct size, improved left ventricular ejection fraction, and reduced mortality.[3-5] The 12-lead ECG remains the "gold standard" for the diagnosis of acute myocardial infarction and the basis for decisions regarding thrombolytic administration.

Recording the Prehospital Electrocardiogram

The feasibility of prehospital ECG recording has been established. Many portable battery-operated devices are available; some provide a recording facility only, and others incorporate an interpretative algorithm that will produce a computer interpretation of the ECG. The ECG can be recorded by various trained personnel. At the Royal Victoria Hospital, the ECG is recorded by the physician who is attending the patient in the mobile coronary care unit.[6] In the Grampian Region Early Anistreplase Trial (GREAT) study,[4] the ECG was performed by a general practitioner (family doctor). Nurses and paramedics[7,8] may also record the ECG in the prehospital setting. Interpretation requires much more training than recording of the ECG. In the study by Foster et al,[8] nurses and paramedics were trained to sight-read the prehospital ECG for the presence of acute myocardial infarction. For those not trained in ECG interpretation, the prehospital ECG may be transmitted to the hospital base station for interpretation by a physician.

The Prehospital Electrocardiogram in Acute Myocardial Infarction

The first ECG recorded in a patient with acute myocardial infarction may demonstrate an injury pattern (ST-segment elevation) or a nonspecific change (ST-segment depression, T-wave inversion, or bundle branch block), or it may be normal. Nonspecific changes and normal ECGs are more common in the prehospital setting than in the emergency department (or coronary care unit) because of the earlier presentation; thus, physicians need to be alert to subtle changes. The value of a repeat ECG after 10 to 20 minutes in inconclusive cases cannot be overstated.

The injury pattern of ST-segment elevation usually is easily recognized and highly specific for acute myocardial infarction.[9] Specificity is almost 100% when a cut-off criterion of 2 mm of ST-segment elevation in two leads is used, particularly if there also are reciprocal changes in other leads. Often, it is more difficult to determine the presence of definite ST-segment elevation in precordial leads than in limb leads, and it is usually possible to be confident of the diagnosis of a lateral or inferior myocardial infarction on the basis of 1 mm of ST-segment elevation in two leads at an early stage. Patients with acute chest pain and ST-segment elevation should receive thrombolytic therapy without delay (Figures 1 and 2). However, the pattern of ST-segment elevation is notoriously insensitive for the detection of acute myocardial infarction.[10] About 50% of patients with acute myocardial infarction will have ST-segment elevation on the initial ECG;[9] thus, half of the patients with acute myocardial infarction will not receive thrombolytic treatment.

The initial ECG in patients with subsequently proven myocardial infarction can exhibit a wide range of abnormalities other than those noted above. The commonest of these are ischemic changes (ST-segment depression or T-wave inversion), left ventricular hypertrophy or strain pattern, bundle branch block, or old Q waves of a previous myocardial infarction.[9] It also should be borne in mind that in a small number of patients with acute myocardial infarction, the initial ECG may be entirely normal,[9] nor does a normal ECG preclude the development of ventricular fibrillation in a patient with myocardial infarction (Figure 3). In exceptional cases, the ECG may remain normal throughout the admission of a patient with documented acute myocardial infarction (documented on the basis of chest pain, cardiac enzyme criteria, and thallium imaging [Figure 4]).

ST-Segment Depression

ST-segment depression and/or T-wave inversion without elevation on the initial ECG is common in patients with ischemic heart disease presenting with acute chest pain (Figure 5). These ECG abnormalities account for approximately one fourth of the patients admitted with suspected acute myocardial infarction.[6] Only a small proportion of patients with acute chest pain and ST-segment depression or deep T-wave inversion are subsequently shown to have acute myocardial infarction; hence, such changes are poor predictors of acute myocardial infarction.[6,9] The sensitivity and positive predictive value for acute myocardial infarction have been reported to be as low as 15% and 39%, respectively.[9]

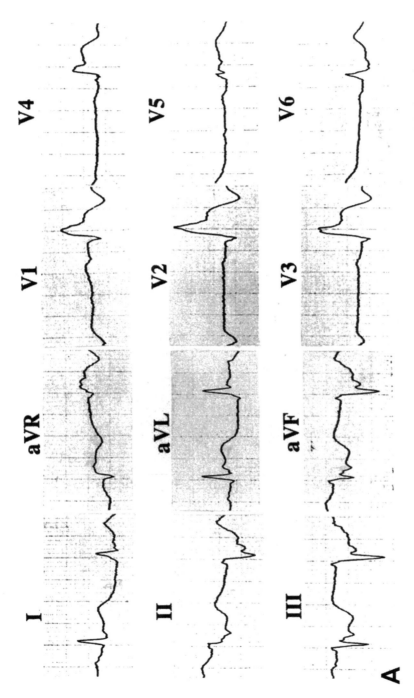

Figure 1. An 82-year-old man and pipe smoker had a history of previous myocardial infarction. He presented with further ischemic chest pain of 2 hours' duration. **A.** The first ECG showed acute anterior infarction with trifascicular block (right bundle branch block, leftward axis, and first-degree atrioventricular block). This usually is associated with a substantially large infarction and a high incidence of complete heart block.

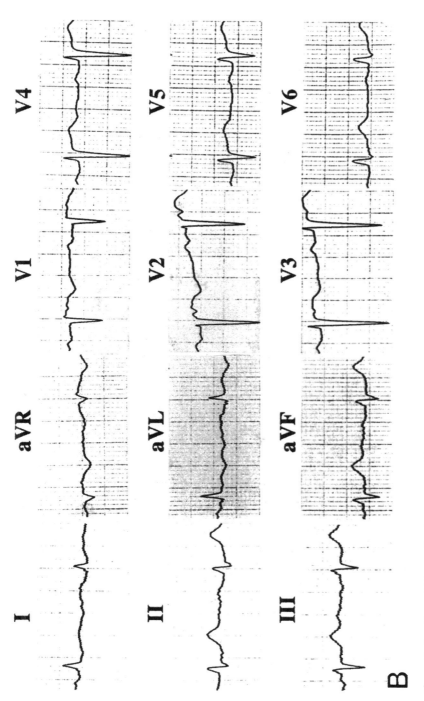

Figure 1. *(continued)* He received treatment with intravenous tissue plasminogen activator, and, (**B**), the second ECG showed that the PR interval normalized and the bundle branch block disappeared with reperfusion. Infarction was confirmed by a maximal creatine kinase level of 4,435 U/L and aspartate aminotransferase of 708 U/L. This case illustrates that early thrombolysis can reverse some of the rhythm complications of acute infarction, including heart block.

179

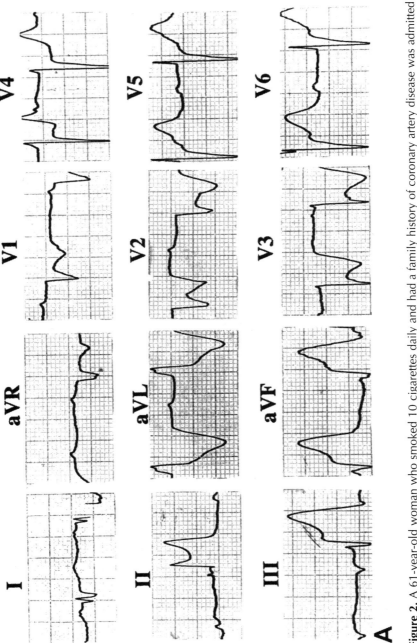

Figure 2. A 61-year-old woman who smoked 10 cigarettes daily and had a family history of coronary artery disease was admitted with ischemic chest pain. The initial ECG was normal. Subsequently, she had a second episode of pain, and (**A**) a repeat ECG showed an acute inferior myocardial infarction complicated by second- and third-degree heart block.

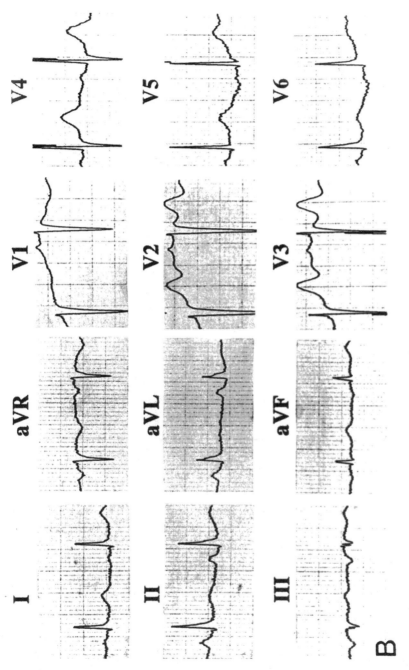

Figure 2. *(continued)* She received thrombolytic treatment with tissue plasminogen activator, and 30 minutes later (**B**) the ECG had returned to normal. There was no subsequent increase in cardiac enzymes. Coronary angiography demonstrated a critical stenosis of the right coronary artery. This case shows the value of repeat ECG recording and the lack of reassurance given by an initially normal ECG. It also shows that early thrombolysis may abort infarction and prevent permanent myocardial damage.

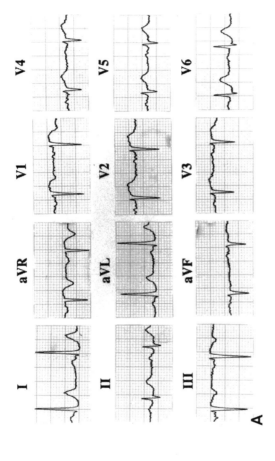

Figure 3. An obese 60-year-old woman with a history of angina presented with chest pain. She was known to have an increased level of cholesterol and a positive family history of coronary artery disease. **A.** The initial ECG was normal. Shortly afterward, she collapsed with ventricular fibrillation and was resuscitated with a DC shock.

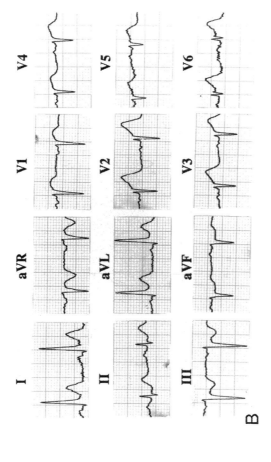

Figure 3. *(continued)* **B.** A repeat ECG showed acute anterolateral myocardial infarction. This was confirmed by a maximal creatine kinase increase of 2,321 U/L and an aspartate aminotransferase increase of 248 U/L. This case illustrates that the ECG may be normal early in myocardial infarction and reminds us that repeat ECG recording is important in patients with chest pain and nondiagnostic ECG findings.

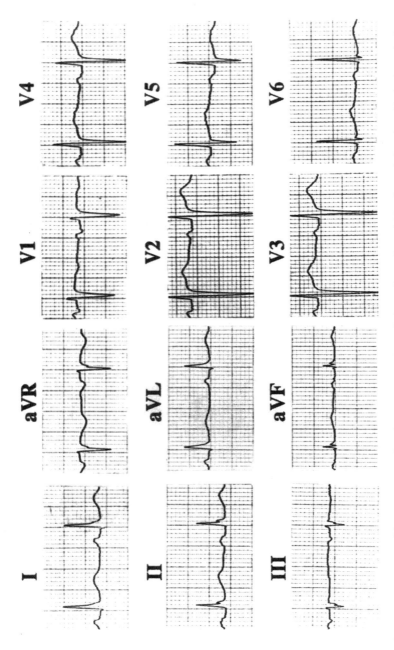

Figure 4. A 62-year-old man presented with epigastric pain and chest discomfort of 90 minutes' duration. He had smoked up to 20 cigarettes daily until 3 years previously. The ECG at presentation was normal and remained so throughout his hospital stay. However, the creatine kinase level increased to 805 U/L and aspartate aminotransferase to 129 U/L. A resting thallium perfusion scan 48 hours after presentation showed a fixed posterior wall defect consistent with infarction. This case shows that myocardial infarction can occur in the presence of a normal ECG and emphasizes the importance of thorough history taking.

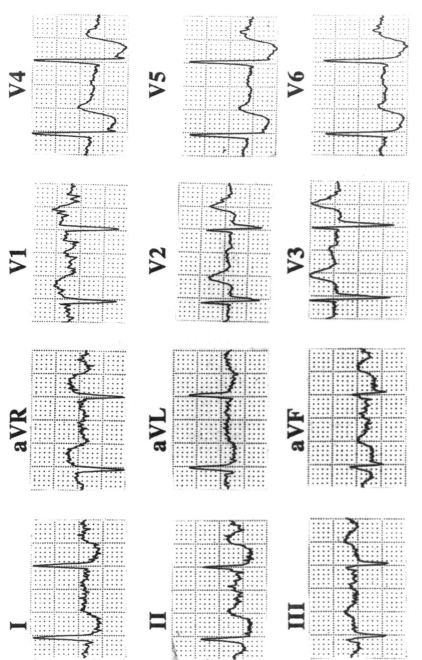

Figure 5. A 63-year-old obese man with hypertension had a history of a previous myocardial infarction. An earlier investigation had revealed the presence of severe left anterior descending and circumflex artery disease. He was awaiting coronary artery bypass grafting. He presented with chest pain of 24 hours' duration. The ECG showed widespread ST-segment depression but no elevation. Myocardial infarction was confirmed by an increased level of creatine kinase (2,626 U/L) and aspartate aminotransferase (314 U/L). This case shows that myocardial infarction may occur in association with ST-segment depression only. This is more likely in patients with multivessel disease, as in this patient.

The consistent finding among patients presenting with ST-segment depression is a high mortality (5-week vascular death in ISIS-2 was 18%,[2] and the 1-year mortality was 26% in the study of Lee et al[11]) whether or not they had an acute myocardial infarction. These patients also have a high mean age and high incidence of previous myocardial infarction.[11] In the ISIS-2 study, no benefit was demonstrated with the use of thrombolytic agents in this group of patients.[2] This may reflect the heterogeneity of the group, and it would seem likely that within the group, those patients with acute myocardial infarction (e.g., true posterior myocardial infarction) would benefit from thrombolytic treatment (because the mechanism is the same as that for inferior or anterior myocardial infarction), whereas those with unstable angina would not.[12] The clinical dilemma is that currently there is no reliable technique for determining which of these patients is having an acute myocardial infarction. Lee et al[11] demonstrated that patients with acute myocardial infarction tend to have deeper ST-segment depression or ST depression in a greater number of leads. When ST-segment depression of at least 4 mm was present in at least seven leads, the specificity for acute myocardial infarction was 93%, but the sensitivity was only 31%.[11] Many cases would be missed using these criteria. Currently, there is no justification for the administration of thrombolytic treatment to patients with suspected acute myocardial infarction with ST-segment depression, except in the rare situation of strong clinical suspicion with very extensive and deep ST-segment depression.

Bundle Branch Block

Left bundle branch block is noted on the initial ECG in 2% to 5% of patients with suspected acute myocardial infarction,[6,9] but the 5-week vascular mortality in patients with left bundle branch block and suspected acute myocardial infarction is 19.8% even after streptokinase, and 14.1% after streptokinase and aspirin.[2] The detection of acute myocardial infarction in these patients is extremely difficult, although it is possible in some patients (Figures 6 and 7). In contrast to patients with ST-segment depression, a definite benefit of thrombolytic treatment has been demonstrated in patients with bundle branch block and acute myocardial infarction.[2]

Various ECG criteria have been proposed for the diagnosis of acute infarction in the presence of left bundle branch block. A recently described, readily usable scoring system incorporates ST-segment elevation of at least 1 mm concordant with the QRS complex; ST-segment depression of 1 mm or more in V_1, V_2, or V_3; and ST-segment elevation of 5 mm or more discordant with the QRS complex.[13] Although these criteria are specific for the detection of myocardial infarction, they lack sensitivity and many cases of acute myocardial infarction would be

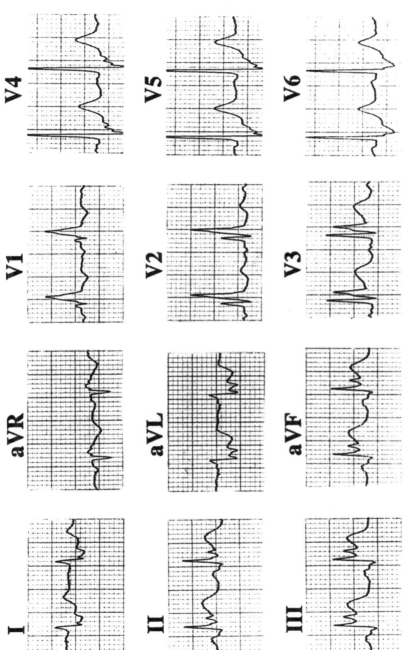

Figure 6. A 70-year-old ex-smoker had complained of intermittent chest discomfort for 6 weeks before admission. He presented with a 30-minute history of typical ischemic chest pain. The initial ECG showed right bundle branch block, with acute inferior myocardial infarction. The subsequent maximal levels of creatine kinase and aspartate aminotransferase were 1,211 U/L and 163 U/L, respectively, confirming myocardial infarction. This case demonstrates that the classic changes of acute infarction can be recognized in the presence of right bundle branch block.

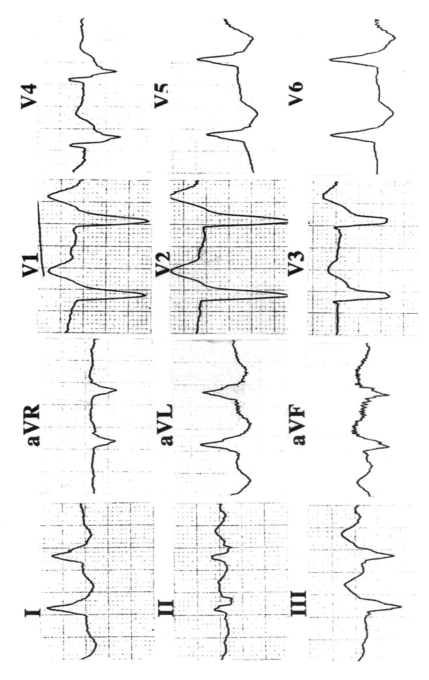

missed. We did not find the algorithm reproducible in our database of patients with left bundle branch block with or without acute myocardial infarction.

Currently, it is our policy to administer thrombolytic treatment to those patients with left bundle branch block in whom acute myocardial infarction is strongly suspected and specific contraindications to lytic therapy are not present. It is our experience that *right* bundle branch block, less frequent than *left* bundle branch block, tends to cause fewer problems than left bundle branch block in the detection of acute myocardial infarction on the 12-lead ECG. Usually, it is possible to be confident of the diagnosis of acute myocardial infarction and, hence, to administer thrombolytic treatment in this situation.

Other Electrocardiogram Patterns in Acute Myocardial Infarction

In addition to saving lives and decreasing time delays to thrombolytic therapy, the advent of prehospital coronary care has enabled the study of the earliest phase of acute myocardial infarction (Figure 8). Some patterns of ECG abnormality have been described and are commonly seen in our practice. In the hyperacute phase, we frequently see the transient development of giant R waves[14] merging with the elevated ST segments and a reduction in S-wave depth (Figure 9). The mechanism of this is uncertain, but it is thought to be an aberration in the propagation of ventricular activation of the region with new ischemic injury. It is our experience that this pattern occurs more frequently in anterior than in inferior infarction. This is supported by Madias,[14] who proposed that this is due to the nature of the precordial leads, which produce ECG records similar to those derived from epicardial electrograms. In addition, Madias noted that the finding of giant R waves is more com-

◀──

Figure 7. A 65-year-old man with no previous history of ischemic heart disease presented with acute onset of shortness of breath due to left ventricular failure. He denied having chest pain. The initial ECG showed left bundle branch block. Ventricular fibrillation ensued and was rapidly corrected with DC shock. It is always difficult to detect acute myocardial infarction in patients with left bundle branch block. In this patient, there was a suspicion of ST-segment elevation in leads I, aVL, and V_6, and streptokinase was administered. Cardiac enzymes confirmed the diagnosis of acute myocardial infarction: peak creatine kinase level, 2,275 U/L, and creatine kinase (muscle and brain fraction), 166 U/L. It is our policy to administer thrombolytic treatment to patients with left bundle branch block and strong clinical suspicion of acute myocardial infarction, because a decrease in mortality has been demonstrated for patients with left bundle branch block and acute myocardial infarction in the ISIS-2 study.

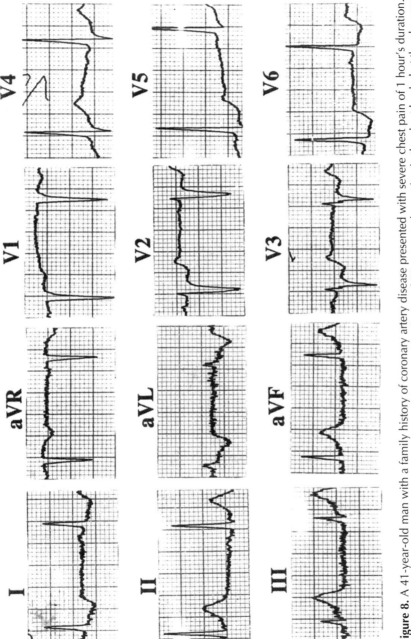

Figure 8. A 41-year-old man with a family history of coronary artery disease presented with severe chest pain of 1 hour's duration. There was early ST-segment change in leads III and aVF, with widespread ST-segment depression in the chest leads, but the changes did not meet the standard criteria for thrombolytic treatment. However, despite standard treatment, the pain and ECG changes persisted, and he was given streptokinase. Cardiac enzymes confirmed myocardial infarction (creatine kinase, 1,178 U/L; aspartate aminotransferase, 148 U/L). This case demonstrates that infarction may occur in the absence of the classic ECG criteria used for administration of thrombolytic therapy.

mon in men, probably because the electrode is closer to the injured myocardium in men than in women. Giant R waves are a marker of the hyperacute phase of myocardial infarction, during which thrombolytic therapy is of most benefit. There is additional clinical relevance in that, in the presence of tachycardia, the heart rhythm may be misinterpreted as ventricular tachycardia.

Another pattern of early ECG abnormality is the hyperacute T wave (Figure 10). These are high-amplitude primary T-wave abnormalities and, as with giant R waves, tend to occur in the very early stage of acute myocardial infarction.[15] It is important to recognize these early abnormalities as markers of impending myocardial damage because treatment with thrombolytic therapy at this stage is of greatest benefit and may even abort the infarction process by early reperfusion of the infarct-related artery.

Improving Early Detection of Acute Myocardial Infarction

Techniques have been sought to improve the sensitivity and specificity of the 12-lead ECG in detecting acute myocardial infarction. Most of these focus on different locations for the placement of electrode leads or the use of a larger number of electrodes. The use of right precordial leads is of value in detecting right ventricular infarction in patients with acute myocardial infarction. Patients with right ventricular infarction have a high incidence of hemodynamic disturbances, sinus bradycardia, and atrioventricular block.[16] A 15-lead ECG system (incorporating a right precordial electrode and two electrodes on the posterior chest) increases the sensitivity for the detection of myocardial infarction without loss of specificity.[17] Of significance is that in the latter study, an increased number of patients were identified as suitable candidates for thrombolytic therapy.

Extensive thoracic sampling lead systems have been used in body surface mapping and have demonstrated that the most diagnostic ECG changes are at electrode sites not recorded by the 12-lead ECG. This has implications for the administration of thrombolytic therapy.[18,19] Technical recording difficulties, time-consuming lead application, and nonstandardized display formats have limited the clinical utilization of such systems, especially in the prehospital setting.

Prognostic Stratification Using the Prehospital Electrocardiogram

The ECG of patients admitted with unstable coronary heart disease may also be useful in early prognostic stratification of patients. Nyman et al[20]

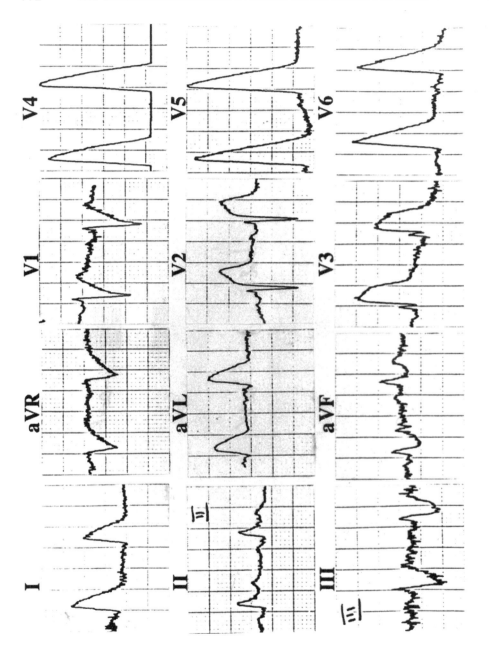

demonstrated that with the end points of cardiac death or myocardial infarction, the 1-year risk for men admitted with suspected unstable angina or non-Q-wave myocardial infarction with a normal ECG was 8%; with isolated T inversion, 14%; with ST-segment elevation, 16%; with ST-segment depression, 18%; and with the combination of the latter two, 26%. Birnbaum et al[21] showed that the initial ECG alone is a strong predictor of in-hospital mortality in patients with an evolving first anterior myocardial infarction. In this study, the patients with tall peaked T waves without ST-segment elevation had the lowest mortality, and those with abnormal T waves, ST-segment elevation, and distortion of the terminal portion of the QRS had the highest mortality. However, these differences may reflect that the former group probably represents an earlier stage in the process of infarction, at which time thrombolysis is of greater benefit in decreasing infarct size and mortality. Prognostic stratification on the basis of the initial ECG may not only guide decisions about administration of thrombolytic therapy but also admission of patients with suspected acute myocardial infarction.[22]

Misdiagnosis

Several ECG abnormalities may mimic acute myocardial infarction and cause diagnostic problems. Early repolarization or high ST-segment take-off is a common normal variant (Figure 11). In uncertain cases, it is helpful to repeat the ECG after 15 to 20 minutes to determine any progression of the abnormality.

Pericarditis generally is considered to be associated with widespread ST-segment elevation, but there are cases in which the abnormalities may be localized, thus causing diagnostic difficulty (Figure 12). Acute aortic dissection is associated with ECG abnormalities in 82% of cases of type A dissection and in 62% of cases of type B dissection.[23] Involvement of the coronary ostia in type A dissection will produce characteristic ST-segment elevation; obviously, the inappropriate ad-

◄───

Figure 9. A 59-year-old man with a history of ischemic heart disease contacted the Mobile Coronary Care Unit after 10 minutes of typical ischemic chest pain. On arrival of the Mobile Coronary Care Unit, after the patient had had 20 minutes of pain, the ECG showed ST-segment elevation in the classic "giant R wave" pattern, with merging of the ST segments with the R wave and loss of the S wave. Shortly afterward, the patient collapsed with ventricular fibrillation and, despite vigorous resuscitation, died in asystole. The ECG demonstrates the hyperacute giant R-wave ECG pattern of infarction that is often associated with arrhythmias and a poor prognosis, as in this patient. Usually, this pattern is seen early in the development of infarction (after 20 minutes of pain in this patient) and, thus, may be seen in early prehospital ECG records.

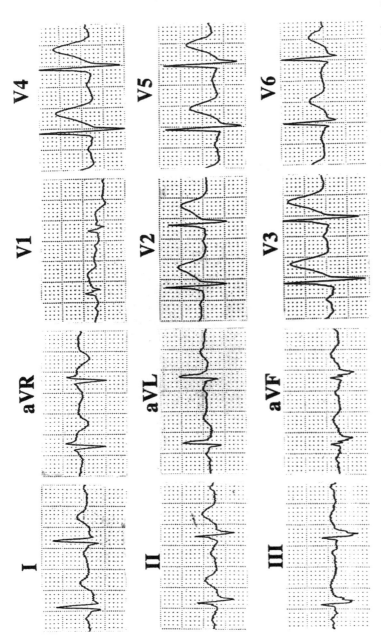

Figure 10. A 66-year-old man with hyperlipidemia and a known family history of ischemic heart disease presented with a 90-minute history of ischemic chest pain. The ECG showed upsloping ST segments in the anteroseptal leads, with tall peaked T waves. These findings sometimes are seen early in the development of myocardial infarction before acute ST-segment elevation. The patient was given heparin and nitrates intravenously, and serial ECGs were recorded to detect any classic changes of infarction that could be treated with thrombolytic therapy. However, the ECGs remained unchanged until 48 hours, when anteroseptal T-wave inversion developed. There was a small increase in creatine kinase to 539 U/L, confirming subendocardial infarction. Cardiac catheterization revealed apical hypokinesis and single-vessel disease, with a 60% proximal lesion and a critical lesion of the mid-left anterior descending artery. This case highlights some of the early changes of infarction and shows that they do not always develop into the classic changes of ST-segment elevation.

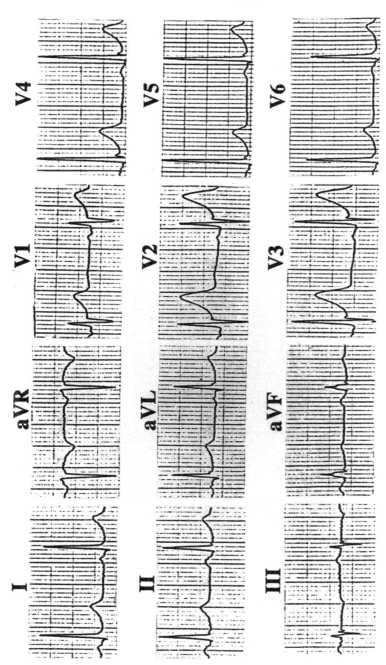

Figure 11. A 42-year-old man smoked 30 cigarettes daily for 20 years and had a family history of coronary artery disease. He complained of chest pain for 5 days and presented after a 4-hour period of significant worsening in symptoms. The ECG showed ST-segment elevation in the anteroseptal leads but no ST-segment depression, Q waves, or T-wave changes elsewhere. In view of this, he was not given thrombolysis. Serial ECG recordings and cardiac enzyme levels were normal and excluded myocardial infarction. This is an example of "high take-off" or "early repolarization," which is often seen in young males. It is not diagnostic of myocardial infarction.

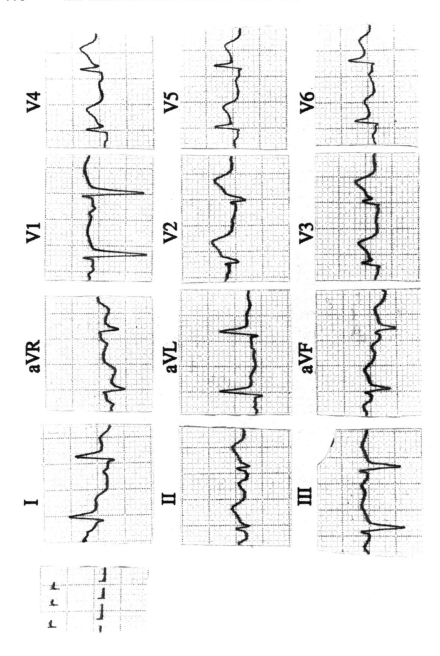

ministration of thrombolytic treatment in this situation may have severe consequences.

To avoid misdiagnosis, the ECG should not be considered in isolation. ECG abnormalities need to be analyzed with regard to the patient's medical history and duration of symptoms. In some cases, supplementary investigations may be required.

References

1. Gruppo Italiano per lo Studio Della Streptochinasi nell'Infarto Miocardico (GISSI): Effectiveness of intravenous thrombolytic treatment in acute myocardial infarction. *Lancet* 1:397–402, 1986.
2. ISIS-2 (Second International Study of Infarct Survival) Collaborative Group: Randomised trial of intravenous streptokinase, oral aspirin, both, or neither among 17,187 cases of suspected acute myocardial infarction: ISIS-2. *Lancet* 2: 349–360, 1988.
3. The European Myocardial Infarction Project Group: Prehospital thrombolytic therapy in patients with suspected acute myocardial infarction. *N Engl J Med* 329:383–389, 1993.
4. GREAT Group: Feasibility, safety, and efficacy of domiciliary thrombolysis by general practitioners: Grampian Region Early Anistreplase Trial. *BMJ* 305: 548–553, 1992.
5. Weaver WD, Cerqueira M, Hallstrom AP, et al: Prehospital-initiated vs hospital-initiated thrombolytic therapy. The Myocardial Infarction Triage and Intervention Trial. *JAMA* 270:1211–1216, 1993.
6. Dalzell GW, Purvis J, Adgey AA: The initial electrocardiogram in patients seen by a mobile coronary care unit. *Q J Med* 78:227–233, 1991.
7. Aufderheide TP, Hendley GE, Woo J, Lawrence S, Valley V, Teichman SL: A prospective evaluation of prehospital 12-lead ECG application in chest pain patients. *J Electrocardiol* 24(suppl):8–13, 1992.

◄───

Figure 12. A 62-year-old woman was admitted with a flu-like illness and central chest discomfort. She was gravely ill with tachycardia and hypotension. The initial ECG was suggestive of acute anterolateral myocardial infarction. Echocardiography revealed pericardial effusion, and the working diagnosis was that of subacute rupture complicating anterior myocardial infarction. Cardiac catheterization subsequently revealed normal coronary arteries and the classic hemodynamic characteristics of pericardial constriction. Because of hemodynamic compromise, pericardial exploration was undertaken; the pericardial sac was tense and thickened and the myocardium itself was noted to be edematous. With further details of the past medical history and immunologic results, the final diagnosis was pericardial constriction and probable acute myocarditis due to systemic lupus erythematosus. The lesson from this case was that the ECG should not be considered in isolation. The clinical history was atypical for acute myocardial infarction; the physician should always bear in mind other, less common possible diagnoses. (Reproduced with permission from McMechan SR, McClements BM, McKeown PP, Webb SW, Adgey AAJ: Systemic lupus erythematosus presenting as effuso-constrictive pericarditis. *Postgrad Med J* 71: 627–629, 1995.)

8. Foster DB, Dufendach JH, Barkdoll CM, Mitchell BK: Prehospital recognition of AMI using independent nurse/paramedic 12-lead ECG evaluation: impact on in-hospital times to thrombolysis in a rural community hospital. *Am J Emerg Med* 12:25–31, 1994.
9. Fesmire FM, Percy RF, Wears RL, MacMath TL: Initial ECG in Q wave and non-Q wave myocardial infarction. *Ann Emerg Med* 18:741–746, 1989.
10. Otto LA, Aufderheide TP: Evaluation of ST segment elevation criteria for the prehospital electrocardiographic diagnosis of acute myocardial infarction. *Ann Emerg Med* 23:17–24, 1994.
11. Lee HS, Cross SJ, Rawles JM, Jennings KP: Patients with suspected myocardial infarction who present with ST depression. *Lancet* 342:1204–1207, 1993.
12. Freeman MR, Langer A, Wilson RF, Morgan CD, Armstrong PW: Thrombolysis in unstable angina. Randomized double-blind trial of t-PA and placebo. *Circulation* 85:150–157, 1992.
13. Sgarbossa EB, Pinski SL, Barbagelata A, et al: Electrocardiographic diagnosis of evolving acute myocardial infarction in the presence of left bundle-branch block. *N Engl J Med* 334:481–487, 1996.
14. Madias JE: The "giant R waves" ECG pattern of hyperacute phase of myocardial infarction. A case report. *J Electrocardiol* 26:77–82, 1993.
15. Collins MS, Carter JE, Dougherty JM, Majercik SM, Hodsden JE, Logue EE: Hyperacute T-wave criteria using computer ECG analysis. *Ann Emerg Med* 19:114–120, 1990.
16. Simon R, Angehrn W: Rechtsventrikuläre Beteiligung bei inferoposteriorem Myokardinfarkt: die klinische Bedeutung der EKG-Diagnostik. *Schweiz Med Wochenschr* 123:1499–1507, 1993.
17. Zalenski RJ, Cooke D, Rydman R, Sloan EP, Murphy DG: Assessing the diagnostic value of an ECG containing leads V4R, V8, and V9: the 15-lead ECG. *Ann Emerg Med* 22:786–793, 1993.
18. Kornreich F, Montague TJ, Rautaharju PM: Body surface potential mapping of the ST segment changes in acute myocardial infarction. Implications for ECG enrollment criteria for thrombolytic therapy. *Circulation* 87:773–782, 1993.
19. McMechan SR, MacKenzie G, Allen J, et al: Body surface ECG potential maps in acute myocardial infarction. *J Electrocardiol* 28(suppl):184–190, 1995.
20. Nyman I, Areskog M, Areskog NH, Swahn E, Wallentin L, and the RISC Study Group: Very early risk stratification by electrocardiogram at rest in men with suspected unstable coronary heart disease. *J Intern Med* 234:293–301, 1993.
21. Birnbaum Y, Sclarovsky S, Blum A, Mager A, Gabbay U: Prognostic significance of the initial electrocardiographic pattern in a first acute anterior wall myocardial infarction. *Chest* 103:1681–1687, 1993.
22. Fesmire FM, Percy RF, Wears RL, MacMath TL: Risk stratification according to the initial electrocardiogram in patients with suspected acute myocardial infarction. *Arch Intern Med* 149:1294–1297, 1989.
23. Hirata K, Kyushima M, Asato H: Electrocardiographic abnormalities in patients with acute aortic dissection. *Am J Cardiol* 76:1207–1212, 1995.

14

Early 12-Lead Electrocardiogram

Correlations Between the Early 12-Lead
Electrocardiogram and the Underlying Coronary
Artery Anatomy and Prognosis in Acute
Myocardial Infarction

Yochai Birnbaum, MD
Samuel Sclarovsky, MD

Introduction

The preferred treatment for acute myocardial infarction is prompt reperfusion by either direct angioplasty or thrombolytic therapy. However, a large number of patients with acute myocardial infarction do not receive reperfusion therapy. Among the most frequent reasons for not receiving this treatment are incorrect diagnosis and underestimation of risk. The majority of hospitals are not equipped to perform primary angioplasty, and many patients have relative or absolute contraindications to intravenous thrombolytic therapy. For choosing the appropriate therapy, especially in these patients, accurate information is needed about not only diagnosis, but an estimation of the size of the ischemic area at risk, the exact site of the intracoronary occlusion, the presence of disease in other coronary arteries, the status of the collateral circulation, left ventricular function, and an estimation of outcome with or without reperfusion therapy. However, to stop the progression of the wave front of necrosis, the decision should be reached as soon as possible after admission. At this early stage, only a few sources of information are widely available, namely, the medical history, physical examination, and the electrocar-

From: Clements, IP (ed). *The Electrocardiogram in Acute Myocardial Infarction.*
Armonk, NY: Futura Publishing Company, Inc. © Mayo Foundation 1998.

diogram (ECG). Data that are collected in later stages of hospitalization, such as the response to reperfusion therapy, peak and time-integral of creatine kinase release, and imaging of left ventricular function and coronary anatomy with noninvasive and invasive methods are not available at this early stage.

Refinement of our ability to interpret the admission ECG of patients with acute myocardial infarction will help in choosing the appropriate therapy immediately on admission. In this chapter, we discuss the information that can be obtained from the admission ECG, in particular, the correlation of the ECG of the acute phase of myocardial infarction and underlying coronary artery anatomy, estimation of infarct size, and prognosis. This chapter concentrates on only the acute phase of infarction (ST-segment elevation with upright T waves) in patients without intraventricular conduction defects.

Shortly after coronary artery occlusion, serial ECG changes are detected by leads facing the ischemic zone: first, the T waves become tall and symmetrical (grade I ischemia); second, ST-segment elevation occurs (grade II ischemia); and third, changes occur in the terminal portion of the QRS complex (grade III ischemia). Although the transition between grade II and grade III is gradual and continuous, we found it convenient for practical clinical purposes to define terminal QRS distortion as emergence of the J-point $\geq$ 50% of the R wave in leads with QR configuration, or disappearance of the S wave in leads with an RS configuration (Figures 1 and 2).[1-3] Only later, the T waves become negative, the amplitude of the R waves decreases, and the Q waves appear. However, not all patients with acute myocardial infarction have the third grade of ischemia (distortion of the terminal portion of the QRS) at admission. Although the underlying mechanism for this difference is still unclear, changes in the terminal portion of the QRS have large implications concerning prognosis, as discussed below.

The magnitude of ST-segment elevation depends on the severity of the subepicardial ischemia. The standard surface ECG is less sensitive to subendocardial ischemia. Subendocardial ischemia may cause either no change in the ST segment or ST-segment depression. However, ST-segment depression may also result from reciprocal changes in leads oriented away from the ischemic zone.[4] Collateral circulation, by decreasing the severity of the subepicardial ischemia, probably tends to attenuate the magnitude of ST-segment elevation.[5] Indeed, in patients with anterior acute myocardial infarction with good collateral circulation, only T-wave changes, without ST-segment elevation (grade I ischemia), may be detected.[6]

The Admission Electrocardiogram and Location of Infarction

Studies evaluating the correlation of various ECG patterns with the location of the infarction have been mainly clinicopathologic, comparing

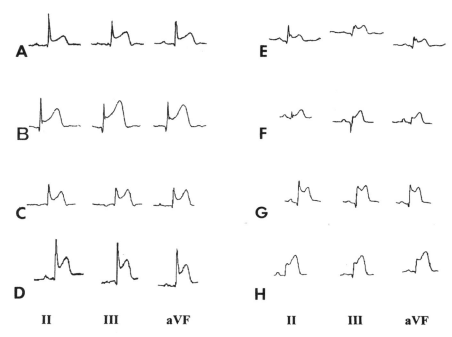

| II | III | aVF | | II | III | aVF |

Figure 1. Admission ECGs of eight patients with inferior wall acute myocardial infarction (recorded at a paper speed of 25 mm/s, at a calibration of 1 mV = 10 mm). **A-D.** Examples of grade II ischemia. The J-points in leads II, III, and aVF emerge at less than 50% of the R-wave height. **E-H.** Grade III ischemia, because the J-points emerge at more than 50% of the R-wave height in at least two of the inferior leads II, III, and aVF.

the ECG of the fully evolved or chronic phases of infarction with autopsy findings.[7,8] On the basis of the presence of pathologic Q waves, an infarct is considered septal when Q waves are present in leads V_1 and V_2; anterior if in leads V_3 and V_4; anteroseptal if in leads V_1-V_4; lateral if in leads I, aVL, V_5, and V_6; high lateral if in leads I and aVL; anterolateral if in leads I, aVL, and V_3-V_6; extensive anterior if in leads I, aVL, V_1-V_6; inferior if in leads II, III, and aVF; anteroinferior if in leads II, III, aVF, and V_1-V_4; and posterior if there are prominent R waves in leads V_1 and V_2.[9] Although anterior wall acute myocardial infarction is diagnosed reliably with the ECG, determining the precise anatomical localization and extent of the infarct is not always possible.[10,11] The standard 12-lead ECG records the summation of the electrical activity of the heart from a distance. Each lead, although facing the heart from a certain direction, is also influenced by electrical events in the adjacent and opponent zones of the heart. Variations in chest shape (especially the

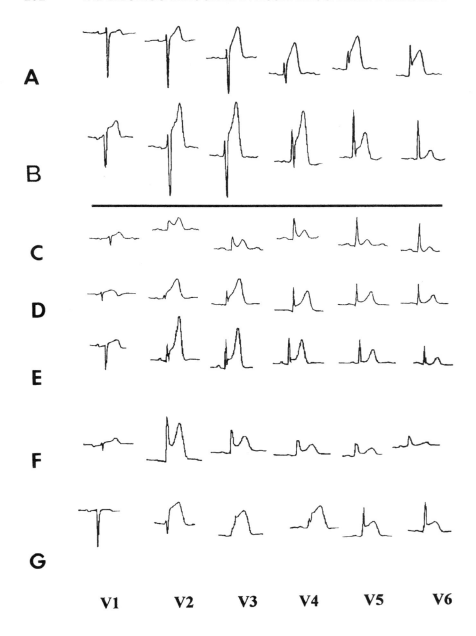

A

B

C

D

E

F

G

V1   V2   V3   V4   V5   V6

anteroposterior diameter), the rotation of the heart in the thorax, the distance of the electrode from the ischemic zone, and the existence of ischemia in other myocardial regions may influence the amount of ST-segment deviation in individual leads.[10] Some areas of the left ventricle, such as the anterior and inferior walls, are well represented by the 12-lead ECG, which is relatively insensitive for detection of infarction in the apical, posterior, basal, and lateral zones, at least in the chronic phase of infarction.[11] It generally is assumed that ST-segment elevation in the acute stage of infarction has the same significance concerning the location of the ischemic area at risk as the Q waves do for the final infarct size. However, no large-scale study has been published comparing regional wall motion abnormalities in the acute phase with the various patterns of ST-segment elevation.

Anterior Wall Myocardial Infarction

ST-segment elevation in the precordial leads V_1-V_4 is considered a reliable marker of anterior wall myocardial infarction due to occlusion of the left anterior descending coronary artery.[11,12] However, right ventricular infarction due to obstruction of the proximal right coronary artery[12,13] and even subendocardial posterolateral infarction due to occlusion of the left circumflex coronary artery may cause ST-segment elevation in these leads.

The correlation of the classic ECG terminology (anteroseptal, anterolateral, etc.) with the anatomical site of infarction is poor.[11] Shalev et al[14] investigated the correlation between ST-segment elevation in the "anteroseptal" leads V_1-V_3 and the location of wall motion abnormalities in patients who did not receive reperfusion therapy. Although hypokinesia or akinesia of the anterior wall was found in 75 of 80 patients (94%) and apical wall motion abnormalities were detected in all the patients, only 15 patients (19%) had abnormal septal motion on echocardiographic examination performed within 24 hours after admission. Only 2 of 35 (6%) patients who had predismissal left ventriculography had septal wall motion abnormalities. These findings challenge the traditional association between ST-segment elevation in leads V_1-V_3 and septal involvement. It seems that this pattern should be renamed "anteroapical infarction."[11,14]

◄───

Figure 2. Admission ECGs of seven patients with anterior wall acute myocardial infarction (recorded at a paper speed of 25 mm/s, at a calibration of 1 mV = 10 mm). **A and B.** Grade II ischemia. Despite having high degree of ST-segment elevation, the S waves in leads V_2-V_3 are preserved and the J-points emerge below 50% of the R waves. **C-G.** Grade III ischemia. Despite having a different magnitude of ST-segment elevation, the S waves in leads V_2-V_3 disappeared in all these examples, and in **G**, the J-points in leads V_3-V_4 emerge at more than 50% of the R-wave height.

Inferior Wall Myocardial Infarction

Although the pattern of ischemic changes in leads II, III, and aVF is traditionally called "inferior wall infarction" and is distinguished from "true posterior wall infarction" (ST-segment depression in leads V_2-V_3), the infarct is in many cases actually posterior.[11]

Posterior Wall Myocardial Infarction

In many cases of posterior wall myocardial infarction, ST-segment elevation is seen only in the "inferior" leads II, III, and aVF. In some patients, posterior wall involvement may be suspected when there is reciprocal ST-segment depression in leads V_1-V_3.[10,15] In some patients, ST-segment elevation may be detected in leads oriented toward the back (V_7, V_8).

Lateral Wall Myocardial Infarction

ST-segment elevation in leads I, aVL, and V_5-V_6 is usually considered to represent lateral involvement. However, leads I and aVL face the basal portion of the anterolateral region supplied by the first diagonal or first obtuse marginal branches, whereas leads V_5 and V_6 are believed to represent the lateral aspect of the apical region. This region may be supplied by any one of the three coronary arteries or their branches. ST-segment elevation in leads V_5 and V_6 may accompany ECG "anterior," "inferior," or "posterior" myocardial infarction. Thus, ST-segment elevation in leads V_5-V_6 is not a specific sign. No one has yet assessed the extension and location of the area at risk in the acute stage of infarction in patients with and in those without ST-segment elevation in V_5-V_6 accompanying acute inferior or anterior wall myocardial infarction. Hence, it is not clear whether ST-segment elevation in the anterolateral leads V_5-V_6 in association with inferior or anterior wall myocardial infarction actually means extension of the ischemic area at risk to the lateral regions or is a pure ECG phenomenon related to the orientation of the heart in the thorax relative to the recording precordial electrodes.

Right Ventricular Infarction

Right ventricular infarction may be diagnosed when ST-segment elevation occurs in the right precordial leads V_{3R} and V_{4R}.[10] However, in some patients who have inferior wall acute myocardial infarction with right ventricular involvement, ST-segment depression in V_{3R} and V_{4R} was found on admission.[16] In some patients with right ventricular infarction, ST-segment elevation is seen in the left precordial leads V_1-V_2 and even in V_3-V_5.[13]

The Admission Electrocardiogram and Coronary Artery Anatomy

There are wide variations in the location and size of the vascular beds supplied by the coronary arteries. In particular, the number, length, and direction of the major side branches vary. The presence of preexistent coronary obstructions with collateral circulation may complicate interpretation even more, because acute occlusion of a coronary artery that nourishes remote myocardial zones by collaterals may cause ischemia in regions not normally supplied by the artery. The surface 12-lead ECG, by revealing the location of the ischemia area at risk, may give a clue to the exact site of coronary artery obstruction. However, because of the variability in coronary artery anatomy, there sometimes is more than one possible explanation for a specific ECG pattern. Moreover, occlusion of a coronary artery in the same site in different patients may result in a different size and location of the ischemic area at risk; hence, the ECG pattern will not be the same.

Anterior Wall Acute Myocardial Infarction

ST-segment elevation in the precordial leads V_1-V_4 is considered a reliable sign of infarction caused by obstruction in the left anterior descending coronary artery.[12] However, in some patients, occlusion of the proximal right coronary artery may result in right ventricular infarction and ST-segment elevation in V_1-V_4.[13,17] Of 79 patients with acute myocardial infarction due to occlusion of the left anterior descending coronary artery, Blanke et al[12] found ST-segment elevation in leads V_1, V_2, V_3, and V_4 in 53 (67%), 68 (86%), 68 (86%), and 60 (76%), respectively. Of 39 patients with right coronary artery occlusion, only 2 (5%), 6 (15%), 6 (15%), and 3 (8%) had ST-segment elevation in leads V_1, V_2, V_3, and V_4, respectively, whereas none of the 25 patients with occlusion of the left circumflex coronary artery had ST-segment elevation in these leads. However, when occlusion of the right coronary artery is responsible for ST-segment elevation in leads V_1-V_4, ST-segment elevation in lead V_1 is greater than in V_2, and ST-segment elevation is seen in the right precordial leads V_{3R} and V_{4R} and, in most cases, in leads II, III, and aVF.

The majority (93%) of patients with infarction of the left anterior descending coronary artery have an "anteroseptal" pattern (ST-segment elevation in leads V_1-V_3).[13] However, isolated ST-segment elevation in the "anterolateral" left precordial leads V_4-V_6 without ST-segment elevation in leads V_1-V_3 is usually due to occlusion of the left circumflex coronary artery or distal diagonal branch and not to the left anterior descending coronary artery. It is plausible that patients with "extensive anterior" infarction (ST-segment elevation in leads V_1-V_6) have a long left anterior descending artery that reaches the cardiac apex and/or larger distal diagonal branches that supply the anterolateral region, whereas patients with "anteroseptal" infarction (ST-segment elevation in leads V_1-V_3) have a short left anterior descending coronary artery or large obtuse marginal branches that supply the anterolateral zones. However, no study has investigated whether there are differences in coronary artery anatomy between patients with "anteroseptal" and those with "extensive anterior" infarction.

Only a few studies have assessed the correlations between the various patterns of ST-segment elevation and the exact anatomical site of the culprit lesion in the left anterior descending coronary artery. The pattern of "anteroseptal" infarction (ST-segment elevation in leads V_1-V_3) is found in the majority of patients with a left anterior descending coronary artery-related infarction, but it is not associated with the exact site of occlusion.[13] No association was found between ST-segment elevation in leads V_1, V_2, or V_3 and a culprit lesion in the left anterior descending coronary artery proximal to the first septal perforator branch.[14,18,19] However, a proximal occlusion of the left anterior descending coronary artery, which carries a bad prognosis, can be identified by two ECG signs: ST-segment elevation in lead aVL[20] and ST-depression in the inferior leads III and aVF.[21]

Lead aVL is oriented toward the basal portion of the anterolateral wall of the left ventricle.[20,22] This area is supplied by both the first diagonal and the first obtuse marginal branches (and sometimes the ramus intermedius artery).[22] In a patient with anterior wall acute myocardial infarction, ST-segment elevation in lead aVL signifies that the first diagonal branch is involved (Figure 3A). This sign is highly specific; however, its sensitivity is low.[20] In a study of 107 patients with anterior wall acute myocardial infarction, Birnbaum et al[20] found that ST-segment elevation greater than 0.1 mV in lead aVL has a positive predictive value of 81% for a left anterior descending coronary artery lesion proximal to the origin of the first diagonal branch. The corresponding positive predictive value of ST-segment elevation in leads I and aVL is 87%. However, the sensitivity was only 46% and 27%, respectively. The explanation may be related to the wide variability in the number of the diagonal and obtuse marginal branches of the left anterior descending and circumflex coronary arteries, the size and location of the vascular beds supplied by each branch, and the presence of the ramus intermediate artery. A greater contribution of blood supply by branches of the left circumflex coronary artery or by the ramus intermedius artery probably prevents high anterolateral region

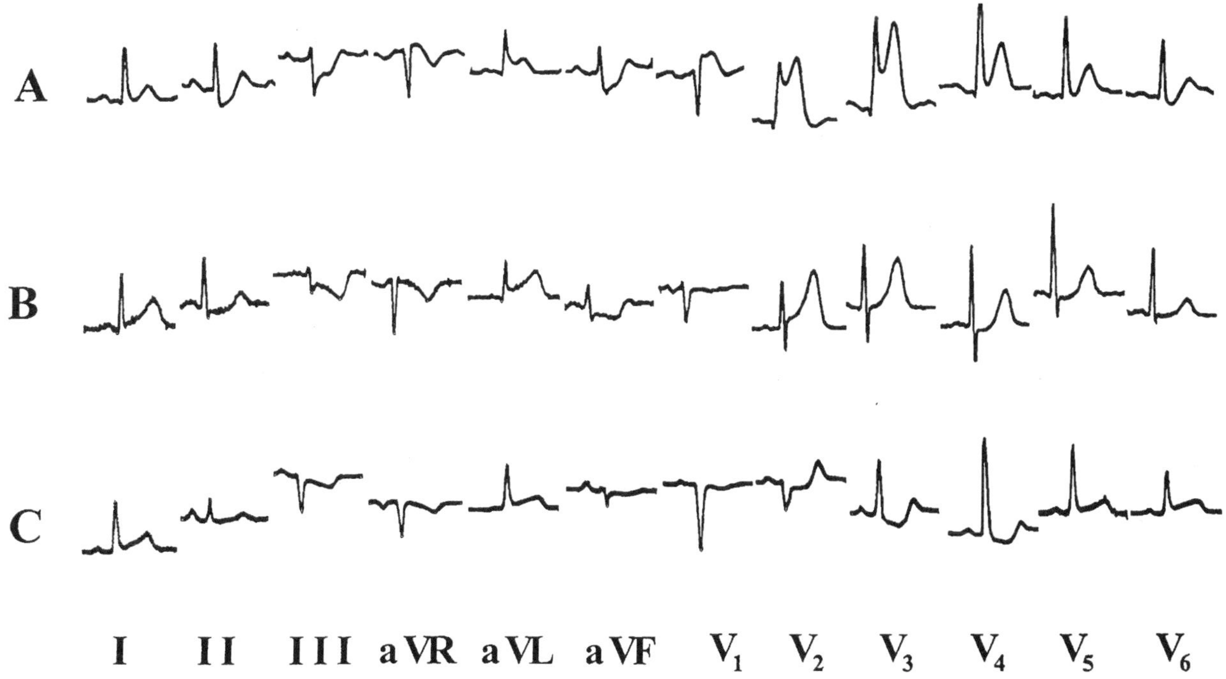

I   II   III   aVR   aVL   aVF   V₁   V₂   V₃   V₄   V₅   V₆

Figure 3. Admission ECGs of three patients with acute myocardial infarction with ST-segment elevation in lead aVL (recorded at a paper speed of 25 mm/s, at a calibration of 1 mV = 10 mm). **A.** Acute myocardial infarction due to left anterior descending coronary artery lesion proximal to origin of the first diagonal branch. Note ST-segment elevation in leads aVL and V_1–V_4 and ST-segment depression in leads II, III, aVF, and V_6. **B.** Acute myocardial infarction due to lesion in the first diagonal branch. Note ST-segment elevation in leads I, aVL, and V_2, and ST-segment depression in leads III and aVF. ST segment in V_3 is isoelectric; there is 1 mm of ST-segment depression in lead V_4. **C.** Acute myocardial infarction due to lesion in proximal portion of the first obtuse marginal branch of the left circumflex coronary artery. Note ST-segment elevation in leads aVL and V_6, mild ST-segment depression in lead III, and ST-segment depression in leads V_2–V_4. (Reproduced with permission from Reference 22.)

ischemia and, thus, ST-segment elevation in lead aVL despite occlusion of the proximal left anterior descending coronary artery. In some cases, ST-segment elevation in aVL may be attenuated by concomitant inferior wall myocardial ischemia caused by occlusion of a left anterior descending coronary artery that either wraps around the apex or supplies collaterals to an occluded right or dominant left circumflex coronary artery.[23]

ST-segment depression in the inferior leads II, III, and aVF during anterior wall acute myocardial infarction reflects a reciprocal response to the ischemia of the high anterolateral region (Figure 3A). Birnbaum et al[21] reported that 21 of 24 patients (87.5%) with ST-segment depression greater than 1 mm in lead aVF had a culprit lesion in the left anterior descending coronary artery proximal to the origin of the first diagonal branch, but only 32 of 98 patients (32.7%) without such depression had a lesion in the left proximal left anterior descending coronary artery ($P = 0.006$). No difference was found between the groups in the prevalence of one-vessel or multivessel disease or significant narrowing of the right or left circumflex coronary artery. They reported a good correlation between the magnitude of ST-segment elevation in leads I and aVL and ST-segment depression in leads III and aVF, whereas the associations between the magnitude of ST-segment deviation in the precordial and inferior leads were weak.[21]

Fletcher et al[24] evaluated 43 patients with anterior wall acute myocardial infarction with technetium Tc 99m sestamibi. They found that inferior wall ST-segment depression does not represent additional inferior wall ischemia. Patients with inferior wall ST-segment depression had perfusion defects that extended significantly farther into the lateral wall in comparison with those without inferior ST-segment depression. Thus, ST-segment depression in the inferior leads during anterior wall acute myocardial infarction is a reciprocal change to high anterolateral ischemia and, hence, another sign of occlusion of the left anterior descending coronary artery proximal to the origin of the first diagonal branch or occlusion of the first diagonal branch itself.[21,25]

The difference between an infarction of the proximal left anterior descending coronary artery and one caused by occlusion of the first diagonal branch is reflected by the magnitude of ST-segment deviation in leads V_3 and V_4. In occlusion of the proximal left anterior descending coronary artery, there is ST-segment elevation in lead V_3 and sometimes in V_4-V_6, whereas in occlusion of the first diagonal branch, there is ST-segment elevation only in leads I, aVL, and V_2, and the ST segment in V_3 and V_4 is either isoelectric or negative.[22,25] In both types of infarction, ST-segment depression is seen in the inferior leads.

Transient right-axis deviation during anterior myocardial infarction with a left posterior hemiblock pattern may indicate significant obstruction of the right coronary artery, with good collateral circulation between the left coronary artery system and the posterior descending coronary artery.[26]

ST-segment elevation in both the anterior leads V_1-V_3 and the inferior leads II, III, and aVF may occasionally be seen in inferior and right ventricular infarction caused by obstruction of the proximal right coronary artery.[13] However, most cases of this are due to occlusion of a left anterior descending coronary artery that wraps around the cardiac apex distal to the origin of the first diagonal branch.[12,23] The high anterolateral ischemia probably attenuates ST-segment elevation in the inferior leads in cases in which the left anterior descending coronary artery is occluded proximal to the origin of the first diagonal branch.[23] Theoretically, occlusion of a left anterior descending coronary artery that supplies collaterals to an occluded right or dominant left circumflex coronary artery might result in a similar ECG pattern. However, none of the 12 patients described by Tamura et al[23] had such an arterial pattern.

Inferior Wall Acute Myocardial Infarction

ST-segment elevation in leads II, III, and aVF may be caused by obstruction of either the right or left circumflex coronary artery.[12] Several studies have investigated the ECG differences in inferior wall acute myocardial infarction caused by either right or left circumflex coronary artery occlusion. ECG evidence of right ventricular infarction (ST-segment elevation in leads V_{3R} and V_{4R}) signifies proximal right coronary artery infarction with a sensitivity of 100% and a specificity of 87%.[10] Bairey et al[27] assessed 12 patients with left circumflex and 29 patients with right coronary artery infarction. All patients had ST-segment elevation in one or more of the inferior leads. ST-segment depression greater than 1 mm in leads I and/or aVL was found in 81% and 33% of right and left circumflex coronary artery infarctions, respectively ($P < 0.01$). An isoelectric or elevated ST segment in lead I was found in all the patients with left circumflex coronary artery infarction, but in only 28% of those with right coronary artery infarction ($P < 0.001$). There was no difference in the occurrence of ST-segment depression in leads V_1-V_4.

Hasdai et al[28] investigated 62 patients with inferior wall acute myocardial infarction. ST-segment depression greater than 1 mm in leads I and aVL was more common in right coronary artery infarction (70% and 100%, respectively) than in left circumflex coronary artery infarction (38% and 63%, respectively, $P < 0.05$ and $P < 0.0001$) (Figure 4). The absence of ST-segment depression in lead aVL was indicative of a lesion in the left circumflex coronary artery proximal to the origin of the first marginal branch. It was seen in 86% of patients with proximal left circumflex coronary artery infarctions, but in none of the patients

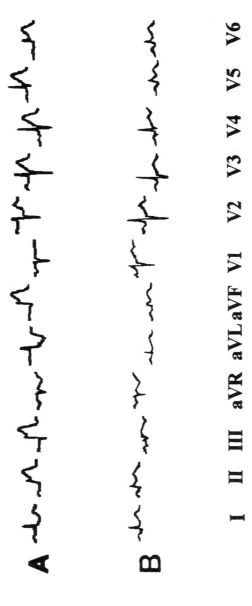

Figure 4. Admission ECGs of two patients with inferior wall acute myocardial infarction. A. With and (**B**) without ST-segment depression in leads I and aVL. (Reproducd with permission from Reference 28.)

with right coronary artery or distal left circumflex coronary artery occlusion ($P < 0.0001$).[28] The occurrence of ST-segment depression in leads V_5 and V_6 was similar in both groups. Thus, concomitant high anterolateral wall ischemia due to involvement of the first marginal branch tends to attenuate the reciprocal ST-segment depression in the inferior leads. Hence, the absence of ST-segment depression in lead aVL is indicative of obstruction of the proximal left circumflex coronary artery.

In the study of Bairey et al,[27] ST-segment elevation in leads V_5 and V_6 was seen in 83% and 24% of the patients with left circumflex and right coronary artery infarction, respectively ($P = 0.001$), whereas ST-segment depression in these leads was observed in 33% and 48% of the patients (not significant). However, because most inferior wall acute myocardial infarctions are caused by occlusion of the right coronary artery, the positive predictive value of ST-segment elevation in V_5 or V_6 for a left circumflex coronary artery infarction is only 59%. It is not clear whether ST-segment elevation in leads V_5 and V_6 accompanying right coronary artery infarction signifies a large posterolateral branch or extension of the vascular bed of the right posterior descending coronary artery toward the lateral aspects of the apex.

The Significance of ST-Segment Depression in the Precordial Leads During Inferior Wall Acute Myocardial Infarction

ST-segment depression in lead aVL is a pure reciprocal change and is seen in almost all patients with acute inferior wall myocardial infarction[29] (except for those with occlusion of the proximal left circumflex coronary artery[28]). In contrast, ST-segment depression seen in leads V_5 and V_6 maximally is usually indicative of multivessel coronary artery disease or concomitant stenosis of the left anterior descending coronary artery.[30] ST-segment depression in leads V_1-V_3 usually is reciprocal to a posterior extension of the infarction,[15,31] is seen equally in right and left circumflex coronary artery infarction,[27,28,32] and is not indicative of concomitant left anterior descending coronary artery stenosis.[31]

Lateral Wall Acute Myocardial Infarction

ST-segment elevation in leads I and aVL is indicative of high anterolateral wall ischemia. If ST-segment elevation in leads I and aVL is accompanied by ST-segment elevation in leads V_2, V_3, and other precordial leads, obstruction of the left anterior descending coronary artery proximal to the origin of the first diagonal branch should be suspected (Figure 3A).[20,22] However, when there is only ST-segment elevation in lead V_2, with isoelectric or negative ST segment in leads V_3 and V_4 (accompanied by tall upright T waves), occlusion of the first diagonal branch is probable (Figure 3B).[22,25] Because of the more posterior location of the vascular bed supplied by the left circumflex coronary artery, when ST-segment elevation in leads I and aVL accompanies its occlusion, there is usually a reciprocal ST-segment depression in lead V_2 (or, at least, there may not be ST-segment elevation in this lead) (Figure 3C).[22] Birnbaum et al[22] evaluated 57 patients with acute myocardial infarction presenting with ST-segment elevation in aVL. Of the 11 patients with left circumflex coronary artery infarction, 10 had either isoelectric ST segment or ST-segment depression of more than 0.1 mV in lead V_2, whereas none of the patients with the left anterior descending coronary or first diagonal artery infarction had such ST-segment depression (positive predictive value, 100%; negative predictive value, 98%). ST-segment elevation of 0.1 mV or greater in lead V_2, accompanied by ST-segment elevation of less than 0.1 mV in lead V_3, had a positive predictive value of 89% and a negative predictive value of 100% for occlusion of the first diagonal branch. T-segment elevation in leads V_2 and V_3 had a 95% positive predictive value and 94% negative predictive value for occlusion of the proximal left anterior descending coronary artery.[22] ST-segment elevation in leads V_4-V_6, without ST-segment elevation in leads V_1-V_3 or the inferior leads, is usually due to occlusion of the left circumflex coronary artery or distal diagonal branch.[12]

The left circumflex coronary artery supplies variable portions of the posterior, inferior, lateral, high anterolateral, and apical aspects of the left ventricle. However, there is large variability in the extent and location of the vascular beds supplied by the left circumflex coronary artery and its marginal branches.[32] The ECG manifestations of acute myocardial infarction caused by occlusion of the left circumflex coronary artery are highly dependent on the exact site of the culprit occlusion, the size and location of the ischemic area at risk, and, probably, additional ischemia due to preexisting coronary lesions in other coronary arteries. Thus, occlusion of the left circumflex coronary artery may produce the classic ECG pattern of "inferior," "posterior," or "lateral" infarction, or a combination of these. However, ST-segment elevation is present in only 48% of the patients with infarction of the left circumflex coronary artery.[12,32] Lack of ST-segment elevation is probably due to the relative insensitivity of the ECG in detecting ischemia or infarction of the posterior, lateral, and apical regions.[11,32] Moreover, concomitant ischemia of the opponent high anterolateral (leads I and aVL) and inferior (leads II, III, and aVF) regions tends to cancel the ECG manifestation of ischemia.[23,28]

The Electrocardiogram Manifestations of Acute Myocardial Infarction Due to Critical Stenosis of the Left Main Coronary Artery

The ECG manifestation of diffuse ischemia associated with critical stenosis of the left main coronary artery is ST-segment depression with negative T waves, found maximally in leads V_4-V_5. Usually, there is no ST-segment elevation or only a minor degree of ST-segment elevation in leads III or aVR (or both).[33]

Estimation of Infarct Size With the Admission Electrocardiogram

Several studies have tried to correlate the final infarct size or the ischemic area at risk with either the number of leads with ST-segment deviation (elevation or depression or both) or the absolute amplitude of ST-segment deviation. However, the results are conflicting. The best correlation between final infarct size (as measured by the Selvester QRS scoring system) and the admission ECG was found using the number of leads with ST-segment elevation in anterior wall myocardial infarction and the magnitude of ST-segment elevation in inferior myocardial infarction (the Aldrich scoring system).[34] However, when this formula was tested against either the ischemic area at risk or final infarct size, as measured with technetium Tc 99m sestamibi scan, the correlation was only weak and related more to the collateral score than to the ischemic area at risk or final infarct size.[5]

Clements et al[35] have also found a weak correlation between the myocardial area at risk (as assessed with technetium Tc 99m sestamibi scan) and either the number of leads with ST-segment deviation, total ST-segment deviation, total ST-segment elevation, or total ST-segment depression. These studies were based on the hypothesis that each lead represents the same amount of myocardium and that a similar size of ischemic area in different locations of the left ventricle will produce the same amount of ST-segment deviation in the same number of leads. However, although the anterior and inferior zones of the left ventricle are well represented by the 12-lead ECG, the septal, lateral, posterior, and apical regions are relatively silent electrocardiographically.

Furthermore, ischemia in opposed regions may cancel or augment ST-segment deviation. For example, right ventricular infarction with posterior infarction may attenuate ST-segment depression in leads V_2-V_3, whereas concomitant transmural high anterolateral and inferior wall ischemia caused by occlusion of the proximal left circumflex artery may cancel ST-segment deviation in leads I and aVL and the inferior leads. In contrast, subendocardial high anterolateral ischemia may augment ST-segment elevation in the inferior leads. Hence, a different coefficient should probably be used for each lead and even for each type of infarction. Moreover, many variables such as the distance of the electrode from the ischemic zone, the width of the chest wall, and presence of collateral circulation have a major influence on the absolute magnitude of ST-segment deviation. Thus, although it generally is true that patients with ST-segment deviation in many leads or a high degree of ST-segment deviation have a larger infarction,[36] the correlation is not linear. Moreover, there are patients with a relatively large infarction who have only minor absolute ST-segment deviation. Early identification of these patients is crucial, because underestimation of their risk usually leads to underutilization of reperfusion therapy.

Birnbaum et al[37] have recently reported an association between distortion of the terminal portion of the QRS on the admission ECG (grade III ischemia) and final infarct size (Figures 1 and 2). They retrospectively analyzed the admission ECGs of patients who participated in the Thrombolysis in Myocardial Infarction (TIMI)-4 trial. Patients were allocated into two groups on the basis of the presence of grade III ($n = 85$) or grade II ($n = 293$) ischemia. The patients with grade III ischemia had a larger infarct, as assessed with creatine kinase release over 24 hours (209 ± 147 U/L vs 155 ± 129 U/L, $P = 0.003$), and a larger predischarge technetium Tc 99m sestamibi defect size ($17.9\% \pm 15.9\%$ vs $11.2\% \pm 13.4\%$, $P < 0.001$). After adjusting for the difference in baseline characteristics, P values for creatine kinase release and technetium Tc 99m sestamibi defect size were 0.023 and 0.001, respectively. Defect sizes of the anterior myocardial infarction, measured with technetium Tc 99m sestamibi, were $24.7\% \pm 16.5\%$ and $18.4\% \pm 16.8\%$ for grade III and grade II ischemia, respectively ($P = 0.035$), and for nonanterior infarction, $11.7\% \pm 12.6\%$ and $6.8\% \pm 8.2\%$ ($P = 0.015$). Creatine kinase release over 24 hours was 280 ± 168 U/L and 189 ± 173 U/L in patients with anterior myocardial infarction with grade III and II ischemia, respectively ($P = 0.003$), and 151 ± 95 U/L and 136 ± 91 U/L in those with nonanterior infarction (P not significant). Thus, the presence of distortion of the terminal portion of the QRS is associated with larger ultimate infarct size. However, it is not clear whether this is due only to a larger initial area at risk or to other underlying mechanisms (such as difference in the collateral circulation or protection by ischemic preconditioning).

Estimation of Prognosis with the Admission Electrocardiogram

A major determinant of prognosis in acute myocardial infarction is the amount of myocardium that remains functional, and this depends on the size of any previous infarction and the present acute infarction. The appearance of pathologic Q waves in leads without ST-segment elevation usually indicates an old myocardial infarction and, hence, reduced myocardial reserves. This is true especially for evidence of old anterior infarction in inferior wall acute myocardial infarction.[38] However, pathologic Q waves in leads with ST-segment elevation do not necessarily mean old infarction or completion of the present acute infarction. Raitt et al[39] found abnormal Q waves in 53% of 695 patients without a previous history of myocardial infarction admitted within 1 hour after the onset of symptoms of infarction. Abnormal Q waves on the admission ECG were more common in patients with anterior infarction.[39] Early Q waves may be only transient and fluctuate or disappear later.[40] In contrast to pathologic Q waves that appear later, early Q waves do not signify irreversible damage and do not preclude potential for myocardial salvage by thrombolytic therapy.[39,40]

Several studies have tried to relate prognosis to either the absolute magnitude of ST-segment shift or to the number of leads with ST-segment deviation. However, the results are conflicting.[3] It was found that the grade of ischemia on the admission ECG (as defined in the introduction) is a strong and independent predictor of short- and long-term prognosis. Birnbaum et al[3] assessed the admission ECGs of 147 consecutive patients with a first anterior acute myocardial infarction (98 patients received thrombolytic therapy). The in-hospital mortality of the 12 patients with grade I ischemia, 77 patients with grade II, and 58 patients with grade III was 0, 3%, and 29%, respectively ($\chi^2 = 22.91, P < 0.001$). Multivariate regression analysis, using the baseline clinical variables available at admission, confirmed that the grade of ischemia at admission is a strong and independent predictor of mortality. The odds ratio between grade II and grade I was 15.6; between grade III and grade II, 11.6; and between grade III and grade I, 181. The predicted probability of in-hospital mortality was 0.002 (95% CI, 0 to 0.027), 0.025 (95% CI, 0.006 to 0.95), and 0.29 (95% CI, 0.19 to 0.42), for grades I, II, and III ischemia, respectively.

Birnbaum et al[2] analyzed 2,603 patients with acute myocardial infarction who received intravenous thrombolytic therapy within 6 hours after the onset of symptoms. Although patients with grade III ischemia had fewer previous myocardial infarctions (15.0% vs 18.4%, $P = 0.02$) and fewer of them had diabetes mellitus (16.9% vs 21.4%, $P = 0.003$), their prognosis was worse. In-hospital mortality for the 1,232 patients presenting with grade II ischemia (ST-segment elevation without distortion of the terminal QRS) was 3.8%, whereas the mortality of the 1,371 patients with grade III ischemia at admission was 6.8% ($P = 0.0008$). The corresponding mortality rates for anterior wall acute myocardial infarction were 10.0% and 4.4% for grade III and grade II ischemia, respectively ($P = 0.0003$). Multivariate regression analysis, using the baseline clinical variables available at admission, revealed that in-hospital mortality was independently associated with grade III ischemia. The odds ratio was 1.78 (95% CI, 1.19 to 2.68; $P = 0.004$). It is important to note that the difference in hospital mortality was seen only in those patients who received treatment more than 2 hours after the onset of symptoms (7.4% vs 3.6% for grade III and grade II ischemia, respectively, $P = 0.0005$), whereas the mortality of those treated within 2 hours was comparable (5.3% and 4.2%, respectively, $P = 0.61$).[2] Patients presenting with grade III ischemia have higher reinfarction rates than those with grade II (4.9% vs 2.8%, respectively, $P = 0.005$). Multivariate regression analysis, using the baseline clinical variables available at admission, revealed that the grade of ischemia present at admission is an independent predictor of reinfarction. The odds ratio was 2.59 (95% CI, 1.31 to 5.13; $P = 0.006$).[41]

In analyzing the patients in the TIMI-4 trial ($n = 378$), it was found that the occurrence of in-hospital mortality, reinfarction, severe congestive heart failure, left ventricular ejection fraction less than 40% (31% vs 21%, $P = 0.07$), as was the weighted end point for this combination (0.21 ± 0.33 vs 0.14 ± 0.28, $P = 0.059$), tended to be higher in patients who presented with grade III ischemia than in those with grade II. Also, there was a trend toward an increase in 1-year mortality for patients with grade III ischemia (11% and 6%, respectively, for grades III and II; $P = 0.092$). One-year mortality for patients with anterior acute myocardial infarction was higher for patients with grade III ischemia at admission than for those with grade II (18% vs 6%, $P = 0.032$).[37]

In inferior acute myocardial infarction, the pattern of precordial ST-segment depression is an equally, or even more important, predictor of mortality. Although in-hospital mortality for patients with ST-segment depression found maximally in leads V_1-V_3 is similar to that for those without precordial ST-segment depression, ST-segment depression in leads V_4-V_6 signifies an increased risk (Figure 5). Hasdai et al[31] studied 213 consecutive patients with inferior acute myocardial infarction (including 100 patients not eligible for thrombolytic therapy). The mortality for the 124 patients with maximal ST-segment depression in leads V_1-V_3 (10%) was comparable to that for the 43 patients without precordial ST-segment depression (12%). However, the in-hospital mortality for the 46 patients with maximal ST-segment depression in leads V_4-V_6 was 41% ($P < 0.0001$). Multivariate regression analysis confirmed that ST-segment depression in leads V_4-V_6 is an independent predictor of mortality (odds ratio of 4.86; 95% CI, 1.93 to 12.26; $P = 0.008$).

Hasdai et al[42] assessed the prognostic significance of the grades of ischemia and the pattern of precordial ST-segment depression at admission. The in-hospital mortality for 38, 76, and 99 patients with grade I, II, and III ischemia was 34.2%, 10.5%, and 15.2%, respectively ($P = 0.005$). However, multivariate regression analysis adjusted for age, diabetes mellitus, previous myocardial infarction, thrombolytic therapy,

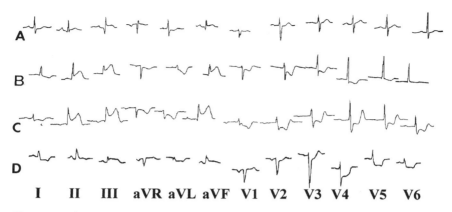

I   II   III   aVR   aVL   aVF   V1   V2   V3   V4   V5   V6

Figure 5. Admission ECGs of four patients (**A-D**) with inferior wall acute myocardial infarction. **A.** No precordial leads show ST-segment depression; **B.** ST-segment depression in leads V_1-V_5. However, maximal ST-segment depression is in leads V_1-V_2; **C.** ST-segment depression in leads V_1-V_6, with equal depression in leads V_1-V_3 and V_4-V_6; **D.** ST-segment depression mainly in leads V_4-V_6.

pattern of precordial ST-segment depression, and grade of ischemia revealed that maximal ST-depression in leads V_4-V_6 was an independent predictor of mortality (odds ratio 4.93; 95% CI, 1.79 to 13.56; $P = 0.002$), whereas the grade of ischemia was not.[42] Thus, in contrast to anterior wall acute myocardial infarction in which the severity of the present insult (manifested by the degree of ST-segment deviation and the grade of ischemia) is the major determinant of prognosis, in inferior acute myocardial infarction, the presence of ST-segment depression in leads V_4-V_6 (which probably reflects diffuse ischemia due to multivessel disease) is the predominant predictor of mortality. Analyzing 31 patients with acute inferior myocardial infarction with ST-segment elevation in only lead III (with ST less than 0.1 mV in leads II and aVF), Hasdai et al[43] reported that the patients with maximal ST-segment depression in leads V_4-V_6 had pulmonary edema or cardiogenic shock six times more often than patients without or with V_1-V_3 precordial ST-segment depression.

Birnbaum et al[44] analyzed 1,321 patients with inferior wall acute myocardial infarction who received intravenous thrombolytic therapy within 6 hours after the onset of symptoms, according to the Global Utilization of Streptokinase and Tissue Plasminogen Activator for Occluded Coronary Arteries (GUSTO-1) protocol. Patients were divided into four groups on the basis of the pattern of precordial ST-segment depression in the admission ECG: group I, no precordial ST-segment depression ($n = 346$); group II, maximal ST-segment depression in leads V_1-V_3 ($n = 700$); group III, the sum of ST-segment depression in leads

V_1-V_3 was equal to the sum in leads V_4-V_6 (n = 162); and group IV, maximal ST-segment depression in leads V_4-V_6 (n = 113). Although peak creatine kinase was higher in group II (630 ± 967, 1,320 ± 1,472, 1,074 ± 1,157, and 902 ± 1,251 IU/L for groups I, II, III, and IV, respectively; $P <$ 0.0001), there was no increase in mortality in group II compared with that of patients without precordial ST-segment depression (group I). Despite having relatively low peak creatine kinase, the in-hospital mortality for group IV was significantly higher (2.9%, 2.8%, 4.3%, and 9.7% for groups I, II, III, and IV, respectively; P = 0.003). Multivariate analysis revealed that in-hospital mortality was independently associated with the pattern of precordial ST-segment depression on the admission ECG. Odds ratio in group IV, relative to group I, was 2.78 (95% CI, 1.26 to 6.13; P = 0.007).[44]

Conclusion

The admission ECG is a simple and inexpensive procedure that carries invaluable information concerning the underlying coronary artery anatomy and estimation of prognosis. Better understanding of the ECG patterns of acute myocardial infarction may help clinicians make decisions about treatment at the time of admission, when only limited information is available. In anterior wall myocardial infarction, ST-segment elevation in lead aVL or ST-segment depression in the inferior leads points to a lesion in the left anterior descending coronary artery proximal to the first diagonal branch, whereas concomitant ST-segment elevation in the inferior leads signifies distal occlusion of a left anterior descending coronary artery that wraps around the cardiac apex. ST-segment elevation in leads V_{3R}, V_{4R}, and V_1 during inferior myocardial infarction signifies occlusion of the proximal right coronary artery, and absence of ST-segment depression in aVL points to an occlusion of the proximal left circumflex coronary artery. Infarct size and prognosis can be appreciated by the presence of distortion of the terminal portion of the QRS (grade III ischemia), especially in anterior acute myocardial infarction, whereas the most important ECG indicator of increased risk in inferior wall acute myocardial infarction is the pattern of maximal precordial ST-segment depression in leads V_4-V_6.

References

1. Sclarovsky S, Mager A, Kusniec J, et al: Electrocardiographic classification of acute myocardial ischemia. *Isr J Med Sci* 26:525–531, 1990.
2. Birnbaum Y, Herz I, Sclarovsky S, et al: Prognostic significance of the admission electrocardiogram in acute myocardial infarction. *J Am Coll Cardiol* 27: 1128–1132, 1996.
3. Birnbaum Y, Sclarovsky S, Blum A, Mager AS, Gabbay U: Prognostic significance

of the initial electrocardiographic pattern in a first acute anterior wall myocardial infarction. *Chest* 103:1681–1687, 1993.

4. Becker RC, Alpert JS: Electrocardiographic ST segment depression in coronary heart disease. *Am Heart J* 115:862–868, 1988.
5. Christian TF, Gibbons RJ, Clements IP, Berger PB, Selvester RH, Wagner GS: Estimates of myocardium at risk and collateral flow in acute myocardial infarction using electrocardiographic indexes with comparison to radionuclide and angiographic measures. *J Am Coll Cardiol* 26:388–393, 1995.
6. Sagie A, Sclarovsky S, Strasberg B, et al: Acute anterior wall myocardial infarction presenting with positive T waves and without ST segment shift. Electrocardiographic features and angiographic correlation. *Chest* 95:1211–1215, 1989.
7. Myers GB, Klein HA, Stofer BE: I. Correlation of electrocardiographic and pathologic findings in anteroseptal infarction. *Am Heart J* 36:535–575, 1948.
8. Myers GB, Klein HA, Hiratzka T: V. Correlation of electrocardiographic and pathologic findings in posterior infarction. *Am Heart J* 38:547–592, 1949.
9. Surawicz B, Uhley H, Borun R, et al: The quest for optimal electrocardiography. Task Force I: Standardization of terminology and interpretation. *Am J Cardiol* 41:130–145, 1978.
10. Fisch C: Electrocardiography and vectorcardiography. In: Braunwald E (ed): *Heart Disease: A Textbook of Cardiovascular Medicine*. 4th ed. Philadelphia: WB Saunders Company; 116–160, 1992.
11. Roberts WC, Gardin JM: Location of myocardial infarcts: a confusion of terms and definitions. *Am J Cardiol* 42:868–872, 1978.
12. Blanke H, Cohen M, Schlueter GU, Karsch KR, Rentrop KP: Electrocardiographic and coronary arteriographic correlations during acute myocardial infarction. *Am J Cardiol* 54:249–255, 1984.
13. Geft IL, Shah PK, Rodriguez L, et al: ST elevations in lead V1 to V5 may be caused by right coronary artery occlusion and acute right ventricular infarction. *Am J Cardiol* 53:991–996, 1984.
14. Shalev Y, Fogelman R, Oettinger M, Caspi A: Does the electrocardiographic pattern of "anteroseptal" myocardial infarction correlate with the anatomic location of myocardial injury? *Am J Cardiol* 75:763–766, 1995.
15. Sclarovsky S, Topaz O, Rechavia E, Strasberg B, Agmon J: Ischemic ST segment depression in leads V2-V3 as the presenting electrocardiographic feature of posterolateral wall myocardial infarction. *Am Heart J* 113:1085–1090, 1987.
16. Rechavia E, Strasberg B, Zafrir N, Mager A, Sagie A, Sclarovsky S: S-T segment depression in right-sided precordial leads during acute inferior wall infarction. *Cardiology* 80:42–50, 1992.
17. Coma-Canella I, Lopez-Sendon J, Alcasena S, Garcia C, Gamallo C, Jadraque LM: Electrocardiographic alterations in leads V1 to V3 in the diagnosis of right and left ventricular infarction. *Am Heart J* 112:940–946, 1986.
18. Strauss BH, Green M: Electrocardiographic prediction of ejection fraction and site of LAD occlusion in anterior myocardial infarction. *Clin Cardiol* 16:213–217, 1993.
19. Birnbaum Y, Herz I, Solodky A, et al: Can we differentiate by the admission electrocardiogram between anterior wall acute myocardial infarction due to a left anterior descending artery occlusion proximal to the origin of the first septal branch and a postseptal occlusion? *Am J Noninvasive Cardiol* 8:115–119, 1994.
20. Birnbaum Y, Sclarovsky S, Solodky A, et al: Prediction of the level of left anterior descending coronary artery obstruction during anterior wall acute myocardial infarction by the admission electrocardiogram. *Am J Cardiol* 72:823–826, 1993.

21. Birnbaum Y, Solodky A, Herz I, et al: Implications of inferior ST-segment depression in anterior acute myocardial infarction: electrocardiographic and angiographic correlation. *Am Heart J* 127:1467–1473, 1994.
22. Birnbaum Y, Hasadi D, Sclarovsky S, Herz I, Strasberg B, Rechavia E: Acute myocardial infarction entailing ST-segment elevation in lead aVL: electrocardiographic differentiation among occlusion of the left anterior descending, first diagonal, and first obtuse marginal coronary arteries. *Am Heart J* 131:38–42, 1996.
23. Tamura A, Kataoka H, Nagase K, Mikuriya Y, Nasu M: Clinical significance of inferior ST elevation during acute anterior myocardial infarction. *Br Heart J* 74: 611–614, 1995.
24. Fletcher WO, Gibbons RJ, Clements IP: The relationship of inferior ST depression, lateral ST elevation, and left precordial ST elevation to myocardium at risk in acute anterior myocardial infarction. *Am Heart J* 126:526–535, 1993.
25. Sclarovsky S, Birnbaum Y, Solodky A, Zafrir N, Wurzel M, Rechavia E: Isolated mid-anterior myocardial infarction: a special electrocardiographic sub-type of acute myocardial infarction consisting of ST-elevation in non-consecutive leads and two different morphologic types of ST-depression. *Int J Cardiol* 46:37–47, 1994.
26. Sclarovsky S, Sagie A, Strasberg B, Lewin RF, Rechavia E, Agmon J: Transient right axis deviation during acute anterior wall infarction or ischemia: electrocardiographic and angiographic correlation. *J Am Coll Cardiol* 8:27–31, 1986.
27. Bairey CN, Shah PK, Lew AS, Hulse S: Electrocardiographic differentiation of occlusion of the left circumflex versus the right coronary artery as a cause of inferior acute myocardial infarction. *Am J Cardiol* 60:456–459, 1987.
28. Hasdai D, Birnbaum Y, Herz I, Sclarovsky S, Mazur A, Solodky A: ST segment depression in lateral limb leads in inferior wall acute myocardial infarction: implications regarding the culprit artery and the site of obstruction. *Eur Heart J* 16:1549–1553, 1995.
29. Birnbaum Y, Sclarovsky S, Mager A, Strasberg B, Rechavia E: ST segment depression in aVL: a sensitive marker for acute inferior myocardial infarction. *Eur Heart J* 14:4–7, 1993.
30. Strasberg B, Pinchas A, Barbash GI, et al: Importance of reciprocal ST segment depression in leads V5 and V6 as an indicator of disease of the left anterior descending coronary artery in acute inferior wall myocardial infarction. *Br Heart J* 63:339–341, 1990.
31. Hasdai D, Sclarovsky S, Solodky A, Sulkes J, Strasberg B, Birnbaum Y: Prognostic significance of maximal precordial ST-segment depression in right (V1 to V3) versus left (V4 to V6) leads in patients with inferior wall acute myocardial infarction. *Am J Cardiol* 74:1081–1084, 1994.
32. Huey BL, Beller GA, Kaiser DL, Gibson RS: A comprehensive analysis of myocardial infarction due to left circumflex artery occlusion: comparison with infarction due to right coronary artery and left anterior descending artery occlusion. *J Am Coll Cardiol* 12:1156–1166, 1988.
33. Birnbaum Y, Sclarovsky S, Strasberg B: Critical left main stenosis (letter to editor). *Am Heart J* 127:1662–1664, 1994.
34. Aldrich HR, Wagner NB, Boswick J, et al: Use of initial ST-segment deviation for prediction of final electrocardiographic size of acute myocardial infarcts. *Am J Cardiol* 61:749–753, 1988.
35. Clements IP, Kaufmann UP, Bailey KR, Pellikka PA, Behrenbeck T, Gibbons RJ: Electrocardiographic prediction of myocardial area at risk. *Mayo Clin Proc* 66: 985–990, 1991.

36. Willems JL, Willems RJ, Willems GM, Arnold AE, Van de Werf F, Verstraete M: Significance of initial ST segment elevation and depression for the management of thrombolytic therapy in acute myocardial infarction. *Circulation* 82: 1147–1158, 1990.

37. Birnbaum Y, Davis V, Sclarovsky S, Kloner RA: Distortion of the terminal portion of the QRS on admission in acute myocardial infarction: correlation with infarct size and long-term prognosis in TIMI-4 (abstr). *Circulation* 92(suppl 1):I-540, 1995.

38. Moshkovitz Y, Sclarovsky S, Behar S, Reicher-Reiss H, Kaplinsky E, Goldbourt U, and the SPRINT Study Group: Infarct site-related mortality in patients with recurrent myocardial infarction. *Am J Med* 94:388–394, 1993.

39. Raitt MH, Maynard C, Wagner GS, Cerqueira MD, Selvester RH, Weaver WD: Appearance of abnormal Q waves early in the course of acute myocardial infarction: implications for efficacy of thrombolytic therapy. *J Am Coll Cardiol* 25: 1084–1088, 1995.

40. Bar FW, Vermeer F, de Zwaan C, et al: Value of admission electrocardiogram in predicting outcome of thrombolytic therapy in acute myocardial infarction. A randomized trial conducted by The Netherlands Interuniversity Cardiology Institute. *Am J Cardiol* 59:6–13, 1987.

41. Birnbaum Y, Herz I, Sclarovsky S, Zlotikamien B, Chetrit A, Barbash G: The admission electrocardiogram: characteristics identifying a subgroup at increased risk for reinfarction (abstr). *J Am Coll Cardiol* 342A, 1995.

42. Hasdai D, Sclarovsky S, Solodky A, Sulkes J, Birnbaum Y: Prognostic significance of the initial electrocardiographic pattern in patients with inferior wall acute myocardial infarction. *Clin Cardiol* 19:31–36, 1996.

43. Hasdai D, Yeshurun M, Birnbaum Y, Sclarovsky S: Inferior wall acute myocardial infarction with one-lead ST-segment elevation: electrocardiographic distinction between a benign and a malignant clinical course. *Coron Artery Dis* 6:875–881, 1995.

44. Birnbaum Y, Herz I, Sclarovsky S, Zlotikamien B, Chetrit A, Barbash G: Prognostic significance of different patterns of precordial ST segment depression in inferior wall acute myocardial infarction (abstr). *J Am Coll Cardiol* 343A, 1995.

15

Prehospital Diagnosis and Management of Patients With Acute Myocardial Infarction Using Remote Transmission of Electrocardiograms to Palmtop Computers

Karlton S. Pettis, MD
Manlik Kwong, BSE
Galen S. Wagner, MD

Introduction

As continued advancement of technology has made possible the development of smaller-sized portable personal computers and electronic equipment, many different applications have been proposed for their use. Cellular telephones and personal data assist devices have become indispensable tools for conducting business of all types around the world, because these technologies give business professionals rapid access to large amounts of information as soon as it is available. With the proper applications, these tools allow professionals to make timely and well-informed decisions, regardless of physical location and time of day. The core technologies, with well-established successful applica-

From: Clements, IP (ed). *The Electrocardiogram in Acute Myocardial Infarction.* Armonk, NY: Futura Publishing Company, Inc. © Mayo Foundation 1998.

tions and histories in the business world, are now being made applicable and available to medical professionals.

Although computers have been used in various capacities for many years in medical centers, there has been delay in integrating them within the clinical environment for direct improvement of patient care. Such tools do not change the fundamental method in which medicine is practiced; rather, they allow medical professionals to practice more efficiently, vastly increasing the quality and ease with which many patient care duties are conducted. The emergency clinical setting, in particular the management of acute myocardial infarction, represents a common example in which the speed and accuracy of diagnosis and care are critical to eventual patient outcomes.

Time to Treatment, Infarct Size, and Mortality

Much time is lost in distinguishing a developing acute myocardial infarction from an acute coronary thrombosis from other differential diagnoses, because this requires the sometimes subtle interpretation of the standard 12-lead electrocardiogram (ECG). For those patients with an evolving acute myocardial infarction, this lost time is critical, because there is a direct relationship between the delay in establishing reperfusion of the myocardium and the amount of cardiac muscle loss. The Myocardial Infarction Triage and Intervention (MITI)[1] trial conducted in Seattle, Washington, between 1988 and 1993 found that there is a clear decrease in infarct size (from 11.2% to 4.9%) when thrombolytic therapy is initiated within 70 minutes after the onset of symptoms. Also, other large clinical trials such as Global Utilization of Streptokinase and Tissue Plasminogen Activator for Occluded Coronary Arteries (GUSTO),[2] and Grampian Region Early Anistreplase Trial (GREAT)[3] firmly established a clinical benefit in mortality rates with reduction of time to treatment. Mortality rates were decreased substantially (as much as 50% in some studies) when reperfusion occurred within the first 2 hours after the onset of ischemic symptoms.

The table demonstrates that the mortality of patients with acute myocardial infarction after the onset of acute thrombosis is lowest when thrombolytic therapy is initiated within the first 2 hours and continues to increase thereafter.[2] GUSTO-I, a large trial that examined overall time to treatment, among other variables, found that only an average of 3% of patients with acute myocardial infarction received treatment within the first hour after the onset of symptoms and that the average overall delay was 2.8 hours at various sites in the United States.[2] Thus, any intervention in this setting that decreases the time to effective treatment translates directly into earlier reperfusion of the myocardium, decreased immediate mortality, and fewer subsequent deaths from poten-

Table 1
Thirty-Day Mortality Rates Defined by Time to Thrombolytic Therapy

Hours to Thrombolysis	% of Patients	Mortality Rate, %	
		Streptokinase	t-PA
0–2	27	5.4	4.3
2–4	51	6.7	5.5
4–6	19	9.3	8.9
>6	4	8.3	10.4

t-PA = tissue plasminogen activator.
(Modified with permission from Reference 2.)

tial secondary complications of acute myocardial infarction.[2–7] Hitherto, many of the studies that have been conducted on decreased time to treatment have concentrated on community awareness campaigns regarding the recognition of the symptoms of acute myocardial infarction, additional training of health care personnel (MITI trial[1]), and prehospital transmission of ECGs to emergency departments using cellular data transmission technology. These studies have shown some success in substantially decreasing overall time to treatment.

Phases of Treatment

The overall time to reperfusion of the myocardium in patients with acute myocardial infarction can be divided into three critical phases: 1) initiation (time from onset of thrombosis until medical attention is sought); 2) diagnosis (time spent distinguishing acute myocardial infarction from other possible diagnoses); and 3) triaging (time spent directing the patient to the appropriate clinical environment for initiation of reperfusion therapy). Several problems exist with the approaches of previous studies to decreasing the time to treatment for acute myocardial infarction as it pertains to these three phases.

1. The initiation phase contributes the largest segment of time (almost two thirds) to the total delay in reperfusion of the myocardium. Large national registries (The National Registry of Myocardial Infarction,[8] and MITI[1]) have found, nationwide, that only 48% to 50% of patients with acute myocardial infarction called 911 or emergency services. Because of these facts, previous studies that attempted to decrease the overall time to treatment focused on the initiation phase. Community awareness campaigns that have used the mass media and have

aimed at hastening the summoning of emergency medical services after the onset of symptoms have met with variable success, presumably because of the limited size and duration of the study.[9] This approach must be examined further to fully assess its effects. Even when heightened community awareness of the symptoms of acute myocardial infarction can get emergency medical technicians involved earlier in the evolution of the infarct (decreased time of the initiation phase), substantial time may still be lost in the subsequent critical phases of intervention — diagnosis and triaging. Here, lost time can offset any time that was saved during the initial phase. In addition, community-based awareness campaigns tend to decrease in effectiveness over time after the program is concluded. This implies that to accomplish a sustained effect, community programs must be ongoing. Continuation requires a source of funding, creates the potential side effect of increasing the number of patients presenting to emergency departments who do not have acute ischemia, and further increases the patient load in some already overcrowded facilities.

2. Increasing the training of health care personnel in the proper diagnosis of acute myocardial infarction can have clear benefits in increasing the number of patients in whom acute infarction is diagnosed correctly. However, all these patients still must be evaluated by an emergency physician before treatment can be initiated. The delay that occurs before this evaluation can oftentimes be a substantial factor in the overall time to treatment in busy understaffed emergency departments.

3. Prehospital transmission of ECGs to emergency departments using wireless technology has been one of the most successful study interventions in decreasing the time to treatment by placing ECGs earlier in the hands of emergency physicians. However, because a certain percentage of patients who have an acute myocardial infarction do not demonstrate clear, classic ECG abnormalities on presentation, physicians who have limited or sporadic experience in interpreting subtle indications of this condition on ECG most likely will need to consult a cardiologist before making a definitive diagnosis and initiating reperfusion treatment.

Remote transmission of ECGs to cardiologists using small handheld, "palmtop" computers integrates many of the benefits of the aforementioned studies, while circumventing the problems inherent in each. It addresses reduction of overall time to treatment by improving efficiency in all three critical phases.

Hardware and Software

The objective of remote ECG transmission is to make critically important information available to the persons most qualified to interpret it as early as possible after the onset of acute myocardial infarction. With regard to the impediments to and characteristics of effective prehospital initiation of diagnosis and treatment, Weaver[9] asserted, "with few exceptions cardiologists are not involved in the prehospital medical care delivery systems. To be successful a prehospital program requires input from knowledgeable cardiologists and emergency physicians. . . . This duty, except in unusual settings, should not be relegated to a less-than-expert physician — it requires an expert in the care of patients with MI [myocardial infarction] and one who is well-read in the continuous refinement of treatment of MI." This requires getting the all-important ECG to the cardiologist who will be responsible for administering reperfusion therapy. To this end, software developers and computer companies have developed programs and hardware for the palmtop computer, a powerful but compact and fully portable microcomputing device small enough to be stored in a laboratory coat pocket or briefcase (Figure 1).

Currently Available Systems

Software applications such as ECGStat (Data Critical Corp., Oklahoma City, OK) that are executed by a cardiologist's palmtop computer are fully compatible with programs executed by the 12-lead ECG. With this system, ECGs are dispatched automatically across cellular telephone lines as soon as they are recorded in the field (Figure 2). After the incoming ECG is screened for quality by an emergency department coordinator, the cardiologist is immediately alerted with a paging tone that an ECG has been received and requires interpretation. The physician needs only to open the palmtop computer receiver to view the ECG. Compatibility of software and programming of the palmtop computer receiver, the coordinator's computer in the emergency department, and the ECG recorder diminishes artifacts and noise in the waveforms and helps ensure that the highest quality ECGs are transmitted.

A slightly different software configuration system soon to be marketed by Marquette Electronics, Inc. (Milwaukee, WI) involves essentially the same process of waveform transmission and differs from the ECGStat system primarily in the method by which the signal is sent. Whereas the ECGStat system uses 30 separate paging signals to transmit an entire 12-lead ECG waveform, the Marquette system uses Internet electronic mail technology to transmit ECGs. This requires only a single continuous radio-frequency signal to accomplish the task. The new method offers the ability to secure this confidential medical data. With electronic encryption and signal scrambling, the radio frequencies dedicated to this purpose can be protected from interception and monitoring by unauthorized sources. The system also allows the emergency department coordinator to confirm receipt of the ECG by the cardiologist. One icon is displayed on the computer monitor (operated by the emergency

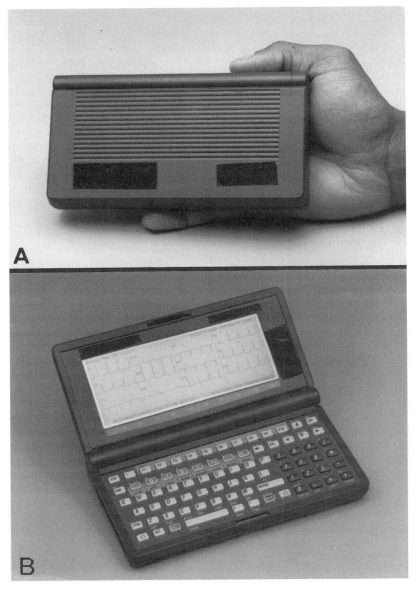

Figure 1. Palmtop personal computer and sample ECG displays. **A.** Palmtop personal computer in hand for size comparison (Hewlett-Packard, Corvallis, OR). **B.** The opened computer displaying 12-lead electrocardiogram. (ECG display from ECGvue program developed by Data Critical Corp., Oklahoma City, OK).

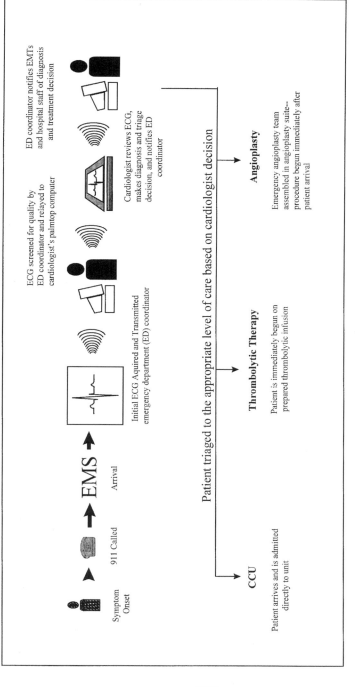

Figure 2. Flow diagram illustrating the sequence of events following the onset of chest pain in a patient in the community. The diagram demonstrates the pathway by which electrocardiograms (ECGs) are transmitted to the emergency department and cardiologist, and the triage decision tree that ensues. CCU = cardiac care unit; ED = emergency department; EMS = emergency medical service; EMTs = emergency medical technicians.

229

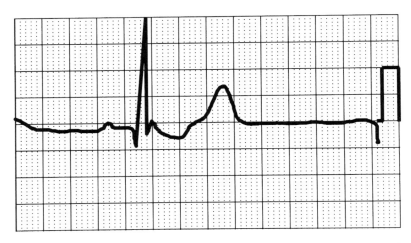

Figure 3. Individual lead display at full resolution (actual size). (From ECGvue, developed by Data Critical Corp., Oklahoma City, OK).

department coordinator) to indicate that the ECG file has been transmitted successfully, and another one is displayed after the file has been opened for review.

Regardless of the method of transmission, a palmtop computer equipped with the appropriate software has the capability to display high-resolution waveforms arrayed in the traditional 12–lead configuration. After the ECG is received by the palmtop computer, the cardiologist also has the capability to enlarge individual ECG leads for even greater resolution, a feature that is useful when making difficult diagnostic determinations (Figure 3).

A typical treatment sequence, in which the emergency medical technicians in the field are trained to operate a portable 12-lead electrocardiograph, is outlined in Figure 2. The ECG obtained is then transmitted by cellular telephone to a coordinating hospital served by the ambulance. An emergency department coordinator conducts a quality assurance review of the incoming ECG for clarity and noise problems. If a poor quality ECG is transmitted, the coordinator has the opportunity to request retransmission or a second ECG. Communication at this stage is through a cellular telephone directly with the emergency medical technicians. When an ECG of acceptable quality is obtained, it then can be dispatched to the cardiologist using the palmtop paging device for diagnosis and triage decisions. It is not necessary that the cardiologist be located in the emergency department or even within the confines of the hospital, so long as he or she is within the cellular telephone service area. After receiving the ECG waveforms, the cardiologist then can make an informed diagnosis regarding the likely presence of an acute coronary thrombosis and triage the patient to the appropriate level of care. This decision involves consultation with the emergency department staff and takes into consideration the availability of given resources. It will entail instructing the emergency medical technicians to: 1) transport the patient to a hospital with a cardiac care unit (patients with acute cardiac ischemia, e.g., unstable angina, abnormal ECG, but at low risk of mortality, or those slated for "soft" rule out for acute myocardial infarction); 2) transport the patient to a hospital where thrombolytic therapy is available (for patients with no contraindication for thrombolytic therapy); 3) transport the patient to a tertiary cardiac care center for emergency coronary angioplasty (for patients at high risk for mortality, e.g., anterior acute myocardial infarction with hemodynamic compromise); or 4) revert to the standard emergency medical services protocol.

After the diagnosis and triage decisions are made, the cardiologist can call the coordinating site to relay the information to the emergency medical technicians and to the appropriate receiving hospital. At this point, the coordinator has the opportunity to select from several appropriate destinations, thereby optimizing resources within a chain of hospitals. For example, assume that hospitals A, B, and C all have facilities to perform emergency coronary angioplasty. The coordinator first contacts hospital A but is informed that all catheterization suites are currently in use. Next, the coordinator contacts hospital B or C to reserve an available suite, and the emergency medical team is instructed to transport the patient to that hospital. Simultaneously, the staff at that hospital assembles the surgical team and readies itself in anticipation of the patient's arrival.

This reduces the time to treatment by: 1) facilitating rapid diagnosis and triage decisions by a highly skilled cardiologist; 2) bypassing emergency department triaging and admission procedures for these critical patients and transporting the patients directly to the appropriate level of care; and 3) notifying the receiving hospital to initiate preparation for intervention (mixing thrombolytic therapy and/or assembling an angioplasty team) while the patient is en route.

Why Transmit Electrocardiograms? The Advantages of Distance Consultation

The aforementioned systems offer several advantages. First, the cardiologist can receive ECG data on the palmtop computer display unit anywhere cellular telephone and paging services are available. (Currently, this area is expansive, with very few areas in the United States and Canada not covered by this technology.) Any subsequent consultation that needs to occur between the cardiologist and the emergency physician on duty regarding triage and treatment decisions can occur over conventional telephone lines or the same cellular link over which the ECG was transmitted. Both of these phases of treatment planning and execution occur much earlier in the process (while the patient is still in the field or en route to the hospital), which leads to a substantially decreased overall time to treatment. Equipped with the ECG before the patient arrives, the emergency department personnel can be prepared to initiate the appropriate therapy without delay. Second, this system makes the skills of highly trained medical center cardiologists accessible to physicians working in rural emergency departments, thereby increasing the quality of care delivered to patients at these sites, while maintaining the freedom of location and movement of the cardiologist. Third, the system can allow one cardiologist to serve as a consultant to several different emergency departments, maximizing physician resources in remote locations in which only one cardiologist may serve a large territory.

Conclusions

The industrial world is gravitating toward greater connectivity. Many countries are using cellular communication as a more convenient, portable method of communicating and conducting business for an increasingly mobile population. Just as cellular communication technology has become a critical tool for business professionals in accessing critical information, so too has it become a valuable resource for physicians. For business people and physicians, the technology facilitates quicker, more well-informed decision making. The use of palmtop computers, cellular, and paging technologies to transmit prehospital ECGs to emergency departments and cardiologists harnesses many of the latest and most advanced electronic systems available to aid in the diagnosis and management of acute myocardial infarction.

The system described allows transmission of ECGs to the emergency department before the patient arrives and facilitates the timely disposition and treatment of these critical patients. In essence, this system is based on the characterization of patients with acute myocardial infarction being similar to trauma patients in the emergency department setting — both are susceptible to high mortality unless effective treatment is administered promptly. Various clinical studies have established the benefits of earlier reperfusion of the myocardium after acute myocardial infarction: decreased infarct size and mortality rate. When used in rural emergency departments that have protracted delays in treatment time for acute myocardial infarction (because of extended transit times from outlying locations, lack of a readily available cardiologist for consultation, lack of cardiac catheterization facilities, or any combination of these), the transmission of ECGs to palmtop computers can provide critical and virtually instantaneous communication links for vital information. In busy urban settings, the system can facilitate the all-important triaging phase, so that patients are not subject to delays from administrative processing. Instead, the patient is routed directly to the appropriate available facility for intervention at the earliest possible time and receives treatment from a team that is informed and prepared for the patient's arrival.

When critical information is disseminated more expeditiously and efficiently, positive effects can be observed. First, overall times to treatment potentially can be decreased substantially. Second, more efficient information systems become key components in the delivery of higher quality medical care at lower cost to both the patient and the health care industry, a priority of increasing importance as the health care industry continues to become more cost-effective.

Future Trends

The integration of computers and information systems into clinical care will most certainly continue, as many technologies originally developed for the lay population for ease, convenience, and efficiency are modified and tested for use in the medical environment. The future will surely see further growth of an industry dedicated to the invention, development, and marketing of computer-based hardware and software for medical applications. Many of these applications are being developed for palmtop computers, because they combine the advantages of being small and portable and having powerful computing and memory capability. Applications for these machines will allow physicians to do more—and to do it faster and easier than ever before.

Cardiologists who are on call and armed with palmtop computers could, for example, carry files with old ECGs on flash disks for all the patients in a practice and access them for comparison when warranted, with the high resolution and analytic capabilities of the palmtop aiding in subtle interpretation and treatment decisions. With the addition of Internet access and electronic mail capability now available for palmtop computers, physicians could also send ECGs instantaneously to other locations, wherever the patient is receiving treatment. Transmitting ECGs in electronic form is superior to the facsimile transmission systems currently used, because it offers greater resolution, confidentiality, and ease of handling. Medical record systems could also be used in conjunction with the aforementioned technology, so that cardiologists could also have the patient's medical record readily available for review or transmission. This would be an invaluable aid to physicians, because it would expedite treatment in acute situations and provide a comprehensive context for the interpretation of ECG data.

These technologies and others being developed constitute exciting advancements in the practice of medicine. As current methods of practice are revised and changed, computer-based technology may offer many benefits not only to cardiologists and emergency physicians but to all health care providers.

References

1. Weaver DW, Cerqueira M, Hallstrom AP, et al: Prehospital-initiated vs hospital-initiated thrombolytic therapy. *JAMA* 270:1211–1216, 1993.
2. The GUSTO Investigators: An international randomized trial comparing four thrombolytic strategies for acute myocardial infarction. *N Engl J Med* 329: 673–682, 1993.
3. GREAT Group: Feasibility, safety, and efficacy of domiciliary thrombolysis by general practitioners: Grampian Region Early Anistreplase Trial. *BMJ* 305: 548–553, 1992.
4. Gruppo Italiano per lo Studio della Streptochinasi nell'Infarto Miocardico (GISSI): Effectiveness of intravenous thrombolytic treatment in acute myocardial infarction. *Lancet* 1:397–402, 1986.
5. Kennedy JW, Ritchie JL, Davis KB, Fritz JK: Western Washington randomized trial of intracoronary streptokinase in acute myocardial infarction. *N Engl J Med* 309: 1477–1488, 1983.
6. Rutsch W, Pfisterer M, Weaver WD, Granger C, Lee K, Ross A: Earlier time to treatment is associated with lower mortality and greater benefit of accelerated t-PA (abstr). *Circulation* 88(suppl 1):I-17, 1993.
7. Martin JS, Novoty-Dinsdale V, Jensen SK, Litwin PE, Weaver WD: Early triage and treatment of the acute myocardial infarction patient: how fast is fast? *J Emerg Nurs* 16:195–202, 1990.
8. Weaver WD (for the National Registry of Myocardial Infarction investigators): Factors influencing the time to hospital administration of thrombolytic therapy: results from a large national registry (abstr). *Circulation* 86(suppl 1):I-16, 1992.
9. Weaver WD: Prehospital evaluation and treatment of patients with suspected acute myocardial infarction. In: Califf RM, Mark DB, Wagner GS (eds). *Acute Coronary Care*. 2nd ed. St. Louis: Mosby-Year Book; 247–254, 1995.

16

The Electrocardiographic Features of Infarct-Related Regional Pericarditis

Stephen C. Hammill, MD
Philip B. Oliva, MD

Infarct-related pericarditis is present at autopsy in 25% to 30% of the cases of fatal transmural myocardial infarction.[1-4] Diffuse pericarditis is diagnosed clinically when ST changes consistent with acute pericarditis are present in leads remote from the area of acute infarction. The clinical diagnosis of regional pericarditis is said to be "difficult, if not impossible"[5]; yet, the regional variety of pericarditis occurs five times more often than diffuse pericarditis in autopsy studies.[6,7] Recently, an autopsy study of 70 patients who died with fatal free-wall rupture after acute myocardial infarction demonstrated patterns of T-wave evolution that consistently occurred before myocardial rupture. At autopsy, the T-wave changes were identified to be associated with infarct-related regional pericarditis and not the rupture.[8] The electrocardiographic (ECG) changes associated with infarct-related pericarditis were further evaluated in 200 patients with acute myocardial infarction without rupture.[9] These patients were assessed to determine the typical T-wave evolution in patients who had reperfusion or failure of reperfusion and compared the T-wave evolution with patients who had clinical pericarditis. The atypical T-wave evolution patterns observed in patients with clinical pericarditis were consistent with the T-wave patterns associated with autopsy-proven regional pericarditis in patients with acute myocardial infarction and fatal cardiac rupture.

From: Clements, IP (ed). *The Electrocardiogram in Acute Myocardial Infarction.* Armonk, NY: Futura Publishing Company, Inc. © Mayo Foundation 1998.

Patterns of T-Wave Evolution After Acute Myocardial Infarction

Typical T-Wave Evolution After Acute Myocardial Infarction

The T wave symmetrically inverts in the ECG leads initially exhibiting ST-segment elevation at the time of acute infarction.[10-12] Typical T-wave evolution involves inversion of the T wave in the leads exhibiting initial ST-segment elevation, with T-wave inversion occurring at 48 to 72 hours after the onset of symptoms of infarction and persisting for several weeks. The rapidity and depth of the T-wave inversion are accelerated by reperfusion.[9] The typical T-wave evolution pattern in patients who have reperfusion is at least 3 mm of T-wave inversion by 48 hours in the leads that demonstrate the most prominent ST-segment elevation at the time of acute presentation. In patients in whom reperfusion fails, the T waves invert by 1 to 3 mm within 72 hours (Figure 1).

Atypical T-Wave Evolution Associated With Regional Pericarditis

In patients with clinical pericarditis[9] or myocardial rupture,[8] two types of atypical T-wave evolution are identified (Figures 2 to 4). Type I atypical T-wave evolution consists of T waves that remain persistently positive for 48 to 72 hours or longer after the onset of infarction in those leads initially displaying ST-segment elevation. Type II atypical T-wave evolution consists of reversal of initially inverted T waves to a less negative or positive deflection in the infarct-related leads 48 to 72 hours or longer after the onset of infarction. Type II changes are also seen in patients with cardiopulmonary resuscitation, reinfarction, or small infarcts as a result of lytic therapy. The sensitivity and specificity of the T-wave changes for diagnosing infarct-related regional pericarditis are 100% and 77%, respectively, which include patients with cardiopulmonary resuscitation, reinfarction, and small infarctions.

The Influence of Infarct Site and Normal T-Wave Amplitude on the Type of Atypical T-Wave Evolution

The type of atypical T-wave evolution depends on the normal T waves present on the ECG before the onset of infarction. Persistently positive infarct-related T waves (type I pattern) occur in 67% of patients with normally positive T waves in the infarct-related leads before infarction

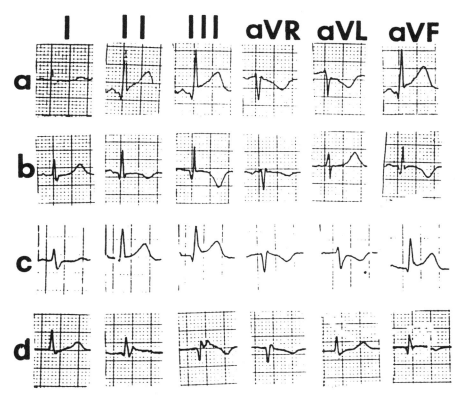

Figure 1. ECGs of two patients with acute inferior infarction illustrating the effect of reperfusion versus no reperfusion on the degree of T-wave inversion 48 hours after onset of chest pain. **a and b.** ECGs of a patient with acute inferior infarction *with* reperfusion and a patent infarct-related artery after thrombolytic therapy. **a.** Initial ECG showing ST-segment elevation and upright T waves. **b.** ECG 48 hours later depicts symmetrical T-wave inversions, with a maximal T-wave negativity of 4 mm in lead III, the lead with the greatest ST-segment elevation initially. **c and d.** The initial and 48-hour ECGs, respectively, of a patient with acute inferior infarction *without* reperfusion. **c.** ST-segment elevation with upright T waves. **d.** Maximal T-wave negativity of 2 mm in lead III, the lead with the greatest ST-segment elevation initially.

(anterior infarct-related pericarditis). Gradual reversal after initial T-wave inversion (type II pattern) occurs in 78% of patients in whom the normal T waves in the infarct-related leads before infarction are less positive or actually negative (inferior, lateral, and posterior infarct-related pericarditis). For example, the normal mean T-wave amplitude in lead III is only 0.4 mm,[13] and 25% to 28% of normal men actually have an inverted T wave in lead III.[14,15] With this small initial T wave in

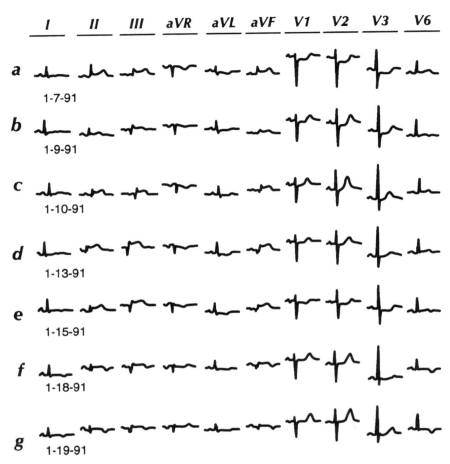

Figure 2. Sequential ECGs of a patient with acute inferior-posterior-lateral myocardial infarction followed by regional pericarditis with *persistently positive* T waves inferiorly and laterally and *gradual reversal after initial inversion* of the T waves posteriorly. **a.** ECG obtained at admission shows acute inferior-posterior-lateral infarction with ST-segment elevation and upright T waves in the inferior and lateral (1 mm V_6) leads and ST-segment depression with a terminally upright T wave in V_1-V_3. **b.** ECG 48 hours later discloses slightly less ST-segment elevation and T-wave positivity inferiorly and laterally, in accord with less ST-segment depression and more upright ("inverted") T waves in posterior leads. **c.** ECG 72 hours after onset of symptoms displays more ST-segment elevation and upright T waves in the inferior and lateral leads than on the preceding day, at a time when the T waves should be more inverted. However, in the posterior leads, V_1-V_3, the ST segments have receded farther and the T waves have, appropriately, become more peaked (i.e., more "inverted"). Pleuropericardial pain and an intermittent friction rub developed in the interim, without reelevation

lead III before infarction, it is not surprising that the T wave usually inverts in lead III after inferior myocardial infarction before the opposing electrical effect of regional infarct-related pericarditis supervenes, causing a reversal of polarity. Therefore, persistently positive T waves frequently accompany anterior or lateral infarct-related pericarditis, because the normal T wave is positive in the anterior and lateral leads. Reversal after initial T-wave inversion frequently accompanies inferior, high lateral, or posterior infarct-related pericarditis, because the normal T-wave amplitude is less positive or actually negative in these regions.

Posterior Infarct-Related Pericarditis

The same T-wave changes occur with posterior infarct-related pericarditis. However, the changes are more difficult to visualize because the posterior leads, V_1-V_3, view the posterior wall with a reversal of polarity. T-wave inversion that would be seen in the anterior or inferior leads will present as upright T waves in V_1-V_3 when the T-wave changes reflect posterior wall repolarization changes (Figures 5 and 6). Because the T wave is normally upright in V_2 and V_3, accentuation of the upright T wave occurs 48 to 72 hours after the onset of posterior infarction in patients who have normal T-wave evolution. This results in peak T waves and is due to subepicardial ischemia. If posterior infarct-related pericarditis ensues, the T wave diminishes in V_1-V_3 and becomes less positive. On the surface, this is at variance with the atypical T-wave evolution associated with infarct-related pericarditis at all other infarct sites where the T wave becomes more positive as pericarditis appears. This discrepancy is explained by considering the upright T wave in V_1-V_3 after a posterior infarction as a "negative" deflection if there was an ECG electrode over the posterior wall at the site of infarction. Alternatively, one can visualize the V_1-V_3 tracings being looked at upside down, and it becomes more apparent that the T waves in V_1-V_3 are "negative" when reflecting repolarization of the posterior wall. Thus, if tall, upright T waves in V_1-V_3 after a posterior myocardial infarction are considered as "negative" deflections, then T waves become "less negative" (or actually positive) or remain persistently positive in the infarct-related leads in all sites of infarction when infarct-related pericarditis occurs.

◀ ──

of the level of CK-MB. Thus, the ECG in **c** suggests regional *inferior* and *lateral*, but not posterior, infarct-related pericarditis at that time. **d, e, and f.** ECGs acquired during the ensuing 6 days. **c and d.** On 1–10–91 and 1–13–91, 6 and 8 days, respectively, after the onset of infarction, the T waves remain upright in the inferior and lateral leads, while the polarity of the T wave has reversed direction in the posterior leads, attaining a minimal "positivity" of 1 mm in V_2 on 1–15–91, **e,** suggesting extension of the pericarditis onto the posterior wall. **f and g.** On 1–18–91 and 1–19–91, the T wave has finally inverted in the inferior and lateral leads, an event that should have occurred 6 days earlier, and has reinverted in the posterior leads.

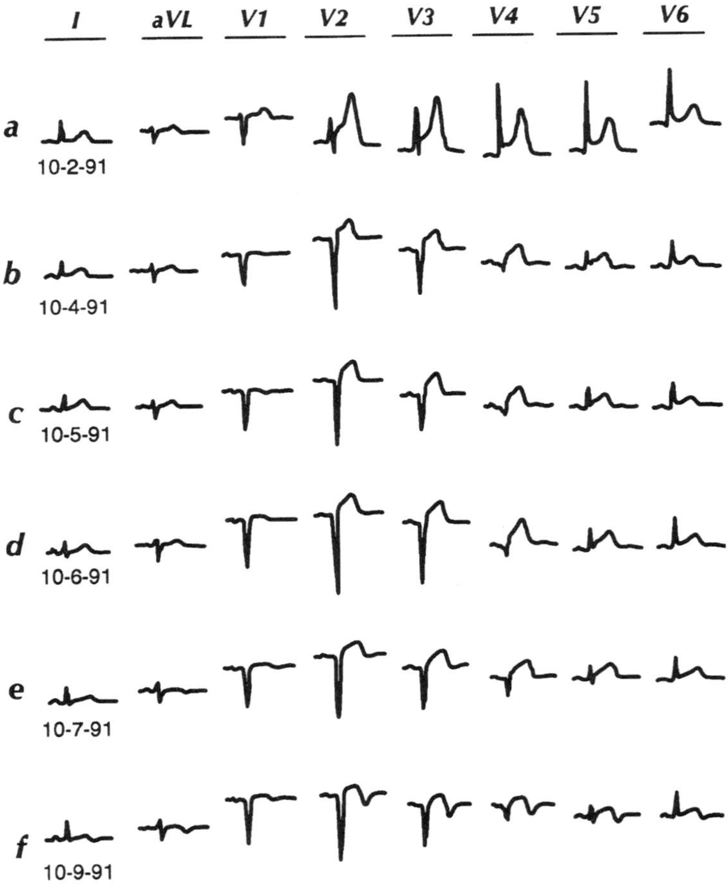

Figure 3. Serial ECGs of a patient with acute anterior-lateral myocardial infarction, with subsequent regional infarct-related pericarditis. **a.** ECG at admission, recorded 2 hours after onset of symptoms, shows ST-segment elevation and upright T waves in V_2-V_6. There may also be 0.5 mm of ST-segment elevation in aVL, using the TP segment as the baseline. **b.** The 48-hour recording discloses *persistently positive* T waves in V_2-V_6. Eight hours earlier, pleuropericardial pain and a rub had developed without reelevation of the CK-MB level. **c, d, and e.** ECGs obtained during the next 3 days as the pericarditis persisted, reveal continued and variable degrees of persistently positive T waves in V_2-V_6. **f.** ECG 2 days after that in **e.** following resolution of the pericarditis, displays delayed T-wave inversion in V_2-V_6 to a degree that should have existed on 10–4–91.

Note the mild T-wave inversion in aVL in **f**, suggesting that perhaps the minimal (0.5 mm) ST-segment elevation in that lead on admission may have been due to a superior (high lateral) extension of the infarction, followed by pericarditis, which resolved and allowed the T wave to invert belatedly on 10–9–91.

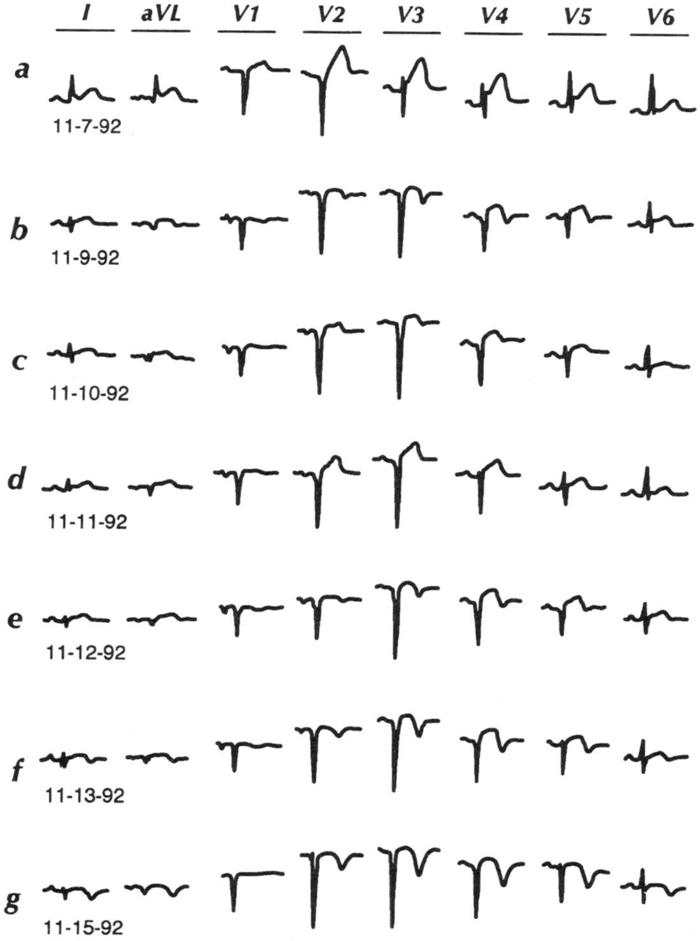

Figure 4. Serial ECGs of a patient with acute anterior-lateral-superior myocardial infarction followed by regional pericarditis. **a.** Admission ECG shows ST-segment elevation with upright T waves in V_2-V_5, I, and aVL. **b.** ECG 48 hours after onset of symptoms (not admission) reveals the expected T-wave inversions in V_2-V_5. In V_6, there is about 0.5 mm of terminal T-wave inversion. **c.** ECG acquired the next day discloses slight, but definite, *gradual T-wave reversal* in V_2-V_6. **e.** ECG recorded as pericarditis waned reveals beginning reinversion of T waves in V_2-V_5. **f. and g.** ECGs after pericarditis had resolved show deeper T-wave reinversions in V_2-V_5 and, now, even in V_6.

With regard to the superior (high lateral) component of the infarction, note the initial (**b**) minimal (0.5 mm) T-wave inversion in aVL, followed by reversal of T-wave polarity to a positive deflection (1.0 to 1.5 mm) in **c, d, and e**, in association with pericarditis. This was then succeeded by reinversion of the T wave in aVL to 2 mm in **g,** after the pericarditis resolved, to a degree greater than on day 2 (11–9–92).

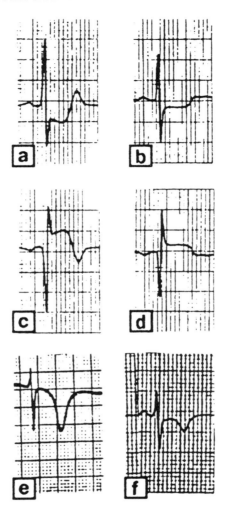

Figure 5. a-d. Four panels comparing posterior transmural (subepicardial) infarction with anterior subendocardial infarction. All leads are V$_2$. **a.** Example of an acute posterior infarction showing downsloping ST-segment depression, followed by a terminally upright T wave. **b.** A subtler example of the same type of infarction, showing a horizontal ST-segment and terminally isoelectric T wave. **c and d.** Appearance of **a** and **b** when viewed upside down. The tracings resemble an acute anterior subepicardial infarction. **e.** Convex downward ST-segment depression and totally inverted T wave in a patient with acute anterior subendocardial infarction. **f.** A subtler example of the same process.

Causes of ST- and T-Wave Changes
in 200 Patients With Acute Infarction

A review of 200 patients with acute myocardial infarction who did not die of rupture identified 43 patients with symptoms or signs of clinical pericarditis.[9] All patients with inferior, anterior, or lateral infarction had ST-segment elevation of at least 2 mm in two contiguous precordial leads. Patients with posterior infarction had initial horizontal ST-segment depression, with a totally or terminally upright T wave in V_1-V_3. In patients with posterior infarction, a prominent R wave subsequently developed in leads V_1-V_3, with an R/S ratio greater than 1. Clinical pericarditis was diagnosed by the presence of typical positional-pleuritic chest pain or a pericardial friction rub. Each patient with pericarditis had T-wave evolution that differed from the pattern of T-wave evolution observed in patients without pericarditis. Patients without pericarditis exhibited 3 mm or more of T-wave inversion by 48 to 72 hours if reperfusion occurred and 3 mm or less of T-wave inversion by 72 hours if the occlusion remained. In 29 patients (67%) who had pericarditis, the T wave was persistently positive 48 hours after the onset of symptoms, whereas in the 14 other patients (33%), the initial inversion that had occurred by 48 hours was followed by gradual reversal of T-wave polarity to form an upright or isoelectric deflection. These changes occurred only in the leads that initially displayed ST-segment elevation, and the changes gradually resolved after clinical resolution of the pericarditis in all except five patients. Three of these five patients who maintained a positive T wave after initial inversion subsequently died, and at autopsy, a localized fibrinous pericarditis was identified. The atypical pattern of T-wave evolution occurred in all patients with pericarditis, and ST-segment elevation receded appropriately in 60%. In the other 40% of patients, ST-segment reelevation occurred with the onset of infarct-related pericarditis in the absence of an increase in creatine kinase (with muscle and brain subunits) (CK-MB) to suggest reinfarction. Patients with multisegment infarctions had T waves that inverted normally in one region but not in others. The area of atypical T-wave evolution was assumed to be the area of regional pericarditis, and in two patients with multisegment infarcts who died, both had pericarditis overlying the region with the atypical T-wave evolution pattern and normal pericardium overlying the region with the expected T-wave evolution pattern.

Widespread ST-segment elevation consistent with diffuse pericarditis was present in only 5% of the 43 patients with clinical pericarditis. Of these 43 patients, all had either persistently positive T waves for 48 hours or longer or reversal of initially inverted T waves. Of the 157 patients without clinical pericarditis, persistently positive T waves were present in 6% and reversal of initially inverted T waves in 16%.

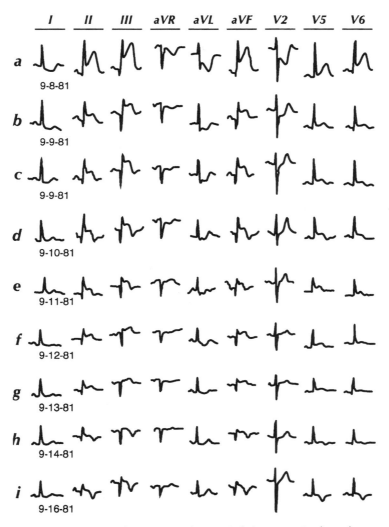

Figure 6. Sequential ECGs of a patient with acute inferior-posterior-lateral myocardial infarction followed by regional pericarditis, with *gradual reversal* of inverted T waves in inferior, posterior, and lateral leads. **a.** ECG at admission shows acute inferior-posterior-lateral infarction, with ST-segment elevation and upright T waves inferiorly and laterally, associated with ST-segment depression and terminally upright T waves posteriorly in lead V$_2$. **b.** ECG 18 hours after admission displays less ST-segment elevation and somewhat less positive T waves in inferior and lateral leads, in conjunction with diminishing ST-segment depression and early, initial inversion of the T wave in posterior lead V$_2$. **c.** ECG 24 hours later reveals a similar (3.5 mm) degree

One half of the patients with persistently positive T waves without clinical pericarditis had had cardiopulmonary resuscitation performed and 85% of the patients with reversal of initially inverted T waves but without clinical pericarditis had reinfarction, whereas the rest had small initial infarcts.

Thus, the other conditions that caused a deviation of T-wave evolution similar to the evolution observed with infarct-related pericarditis were cardiopulmonary resuscitation, reinfarction, and very small infarcts. Small infarcts can be differentiated from pericarditis because they are usually associated with minimal or no QRS changes and only a small increase in the level of CK-MB. With infarct-related pericarditis, the infarctions were usually large, with definite QRS changes and a peak CK-MB greater than 50 IU/L. Reinfarction was associated with abrupt T-wave changes at the time of the new chest pain, whereas the T-wave changes associated with pericarditis developed gradually over several hours to days. By paying careful attention to the T-wave pattern on serial ECGs or monitoring strips, the gradual nature of atypical T-wave evolution associated with infarct-related pericarditis can be observed.

Pathophysiologic Causes of Regional Infarct-Related Pericarditis

The persistently positive T waves and reversal of initially inverted T waves are ECG expressions of similar pathophysiologic processes. Dur-

◄——————————————————————————————

of ST-segment and T-wave elevation in II, III, and aVF, but with beginning terminal negativity of the T wave, most evident in lead III. In V_5 and V_6, the T wave has minimally inverted terminally, while in V_2, the T wave is slightly more peaked (inverted) than on the preceding day. **d.** ECG 2 days after admission depicts less ST-segment elevation and inversion of the T wave in lead III to 3 mm and 0.5 to 1.0 mm in V_5 and V_6 terminally. In V_2, the T wave has peaked (inverted) to a maximum of 8 mm. This represents the expected T-wave response 48 hours after onset of acute myocardial infarction. **e.** ECG obtained the following day after the development of positional-pleuritic pain and pericardial rub discloses *gradual reversal* of T-wave polarity in inferior-posterior and lateral leads without reelevation of the ST segment or CK-MB level. The T wave is now positive, except for a 0.5-mm terminal negative deflection in lead III. **f.** ECG recorded the next day as signs and symptoms of pericarditis continued shows accentuation of the T wave to a maximum of 4 mm in lead III and reduction of T-wave amplitude to 2 mm in lead V_2 (reflecting the posterior regional pericarditis). **g.** ECG obtained the following day displays gradual resolution of both the ST-segment elevation and T-wave positivity in inferior and lateral leads as pericarditis wanes. **h.** ECG recorded on the sixth day shows reinversion of inferior T waves and early reinversion of lateral and posterior T waves after resolution of the pericarditis. The degree of reinversion on day 6 is comparable to that on day 2 (**b**), whereas the degree of ST-segment elevation is less marked. **i.** ECG on the next day reveals even deeper T-wave inversion in all three regions.

ing pericarditis, the ECG initially demonstrates ST-segment elevation, with upright T waves.[16] These changes are believed to be due to subepicardial inflammation.[16-19] When the ECG changes occur after myocardial infarction, they most likely indicate that the necrotic front has reached the subepicardial myocardium. Inverted T waves overlying the infarct zone reflect subepicardial ischemia due to asynchronous repolarization created by delayed depolarization within the ischemic subepicardial zone.[20,21] When this layer becomes necrotic, more synchronous repolarization may ensue, which will result in either persistently positive T waves or reversal of inverted T waves, depending on how quickly the necrotic process reaches the subepicardial myocardium. The T-wave alterations associated with infarct-related pericarditis are similar to those observed more than 50 years ago by Burchell and colleagues,[22] when acute myocardial infarction was associated with local pericarditis in the dog.

Monitoring-Lead Protocol

A protocol to help differentiate among recurrent angina, reinfarction, and infarct-related regional pericarditis is shown in Table 1. This algo-

---

Table 1
Protocol for Following T-Wave Evolution After Acute Myocardial Infarction

1. Determine the single lead on the standard 12-lead body surface admission ECG that displays the most ST-segment elevation and select it as the primary monitor lead. This permits the detection of both recurrent ischemia/injury within the region of infarction and regional infarct-related pericarditis.
2. Select a lead that shows no ST-segment elevation on the admission ECG and establish it as a second monitor lead to detect ischemia at a distance. At least one of the two monitor leads should also have good P-wave morphology for assessment of cardiac arrhythmias.
3. Set the gain at 1 cm = 1 mV. Do not change the polarity or gain of the lead subsequently.
4. Record at 25 mm/s, and mount monitor strips every 8 hr and if recurrent chest pain occurs.
5. Obtain STAT 12-lead ECG before administering nitroglycerin for recurrent chest pain.
6. Query patient about characteristics of recurrent chest pain, e.g., quality, location, radiation, relationship to position and/or respiration. Listen for pericardial friction rub.
7. Review the serial monitor strips and 12-lead ECGs to determine if the T wave has become abruptly upright (implying reinfarction or angina "pseudonormalization of an inverted T wave") or gradually upright (implying regional post-infarct-related pericarditis). Or has it remained persistently positive (also implying regional infarct-related pericarditis)?

---

rithm permits the detection of ischemia within the area of infarction, ischemia at a distance, reinfarction, and infarct-related regional pericarditis. After the appropriate monitor lead that reflects the area of infarction is selected, it is important that the polarity and gain of the lead not be changed. This protocol is not applicable in the presence of electrolyte disturbances, type 1-A antiarrhythmic drugs, or right or left bundle branch block.

Summary and Clinical Implications

Both the speed and the depth of T-wave inversion depend on whether reperfusion of the infarcted myocardium occurs. With reperfusion, the maximal T-wave negativity of 3 mm or more is attained within 48 hours after the onset of infarction. In the absence of reperfusion, the process is delayed to 72 hours and the maximal T-wave negativity is between 1 and 3 mm. Once inverted, the T wave should not reinvert for several weeks after infarction. When infarct-related pericarditis follows infarction, there is departure from this normal T-wave evolution. The T waves either remain persistently positive after 48 to 72 hours or demonstrate gradual, premature reversal of initially inverted T waves. These T-wave changes can be quite misleading and deceptive, because they make the ECG look more "normal." The T-wave changes present in infarct-related pericarditis are accompanied by persistent, progressive, or recurrent ST-segment elevation in only 40% of patients. The ST-segment changes presumably are also due to the overlying regional pericarditis. The T-wave changes are more consistent and easier to identify than the ST-segment changes, because the T-wave alterations are directional, whereas the ST-segment alterations are magnitudinal. Widespread ST-segment elevation, a time-honored sign of diffuse pericarditis, is not commonly present. Identification of patients with recurrent chest pain caused by infarct-related pericarditis (Table 2) will improve patient care

Table 2
Causes of Postinfarction Chest Pain in 200 Patients With Acute Myocardial Infarction

	Patients, %	
Cause	*Without Lytic Therapy* (n = 85)	*With Lytic Therapy* (n = 115)
Pericarditis	30	15
Postinfarction angina	13	15
Reinfarction	6	15

and avoid the expense and problems that occur if the pain is misdiagnosed as recurrent angina or recurrent infarction, both of which should be associated with rapid changes in the ST segment and T waves, in contrast to the slower T-wave changes of infarct-related pericarditis.

References

1. Erhardt LR: Clinical and pathological observations in different types of acute myocardial infarction. *Acta Med Scand* (suppl)560:1–78, 1974.
2. Wang CH, Bland EF, White PD: A note on coronary occlusion and myocardial infarction found post mortem at the Massachusetts General Hospital during the twenty-year period from 1926 to 1945 inclusive. *Ann Intern Med* 29:601–606, 1948.
3. Appelbaum E, Nicolson GHB: Occlusive diseases of the coronary arteries: an analysis of the pathological anatomy in one hundred sixty-eight cases, with electrocardiographic correlation in thirty-six of these. *Am Heart J* 10:660–680, 1934–1935.
4. Roeske WR, Savage RM, O'Rourke RA, Bloor CM: Clinicopathologic correlations in patients after myocardial infarction. *Circulation* 63:36–45, 1981.
5. Likoff W: Pericarditis complicating myocardial infarction. *Am J Cardiol* 7:69–72, 1961.
6. Langendorf R: Effect of diffuse pericarditis on electrocardiographic pattern of recent myocardial infarction. *Am Heart J* 22:86–104, 1941.
7. Stewart CF, Turner KB: Note on pericardial involvement in coronary thrombosis. *Am Heart J* 15:232–234, 1938.
8. Oliva PB, Hammill SC, Edwards WD: Cardiac rupture, a clinically predictable complication of acute myocardial infarction: report of 70 cases with clinicopathologic correlations. *J Am Coll Cardiol* 22:720–726, 1993.
9. Oliva PB, Hammill SC, Edwards WD: Electrocardiographic diagnosis of postinfarction regional pericarditis. Ancillary observations regarding the effect of reperfusion on the rapidity and amplitude of T wave inversion after acute myocardial infarction. *Circulation* 88:896–904, 1993.
10. Smith FM: Electrocardiographic changes following occlusion of left coronary artery. *Arch Intern Med* 32:497–509, 1923.
11. Parkinson J, Bedford DE: Successive changes in electrocardiogram after cardiac infarction (coronary thrombosis). *Heart* 14:195–239, 1928.
12. Pardee HEB: An electrocardiographic sign of coronary artery obstruction. *Arch Intern Med* 26:244–257, 1920.
13. Lepeschkin E: Duration of electrocardiographic deflections and intervals: man. Part II. Tabular. In: Altman PL, Dittmer DS (eds). *Respiration and Circulation.* Bethesda, MD: Federation of American Societies for Experimental Biology; 277–278, 1971.
14. Stewart CB, Manning GW: Detailed analysis of electrocardiograms of 500 R.C.A.F. aircrew. *Am Heart J* 27:502–523, 1944.
15. Graybiel A, McFarland RA, Gates D, Webster FA: Analysis of electrocardiograms obtained from 1,000 young healthy aviators. *Am Heart J* 27:524–549, 1944.
16. Spodick DH: *Acute Pericarditis.* New York: Grune & Stratton; 1959.
17. Shabetai R: *The Pericardium.* New York: Grune & Stratton; 391–397, 1981.
18. Spodick DH: Electrocardiographic changes in acute pericarditis. In: Fowler NO

(ed). *The Pericardium in Health and Disease.* Mount Kisco, NY: Futura Publishing Co., Inc.; 92, 1985.

19. Surawicz B, Lasseter KC: Electrocardiogram in pericarditis. *Am J Cardiol* 26: 471–474, 1970.
20. Horan LG, Flowers NC: Electrocardiography and vectorcardiography. In: Braunwald E (ed). *Heart Disease: A Textbook of Cardiovascular Medicine.* Vol. 1. Philadelphia: WB Saunders; 234, 1980.
21. Elharrar V, Zipes DP: Cardiac electrophysiologic alterations during myocardial ischemia. *Am J Physiol* 233:H329-H345, 1977.
22. Burchell HB, Barnes AR, Mann FC: Electrocardiographic picture of experimental localized pericarditis. *Am Heart J* 18:133–144, 1939.

Index